Teens, Screens, and Social Connection

Alma Spaniardi • Janki Modi Avari
Editors

Teens, Screens, and Social Connection

An Evidence-Based Guide to Key Problems and Solutions

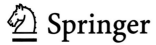

Editors
Alma Spaniardi
Department of Child and Adolescent
Psychiatry
Weill Cornell Medicine
New York-Presbyterian
New York, NY, USA

Janki Modi Avari
Office of Mental Health-New York City
Children's Center
New York, NY, USA

ISBN 978-3-031-24803-0   ISBN 978-3-031-24804-7   (eBook)
https://doi.org/10.1007/978-3-031-24804-7

© The Editor(s) (if applicable) and The Author(s), under exclusive license to Springer Nature
Switzerland AG 2023
This work is subject to copyright. All rights are solely and exclusively licensed by the Publisher, whether
the whole or part of the material is concerned, specifically the rights of translation, reprinting, reuse of
illustrations, recitation, broadcasting, reproduction on microfilms or in any other physical way, and transmission or information storage and retrieval, electronic adaptation, computer software, or by similar or
dissimilar methodology now known or hereafter developed.
The use of general descriptive names, registered names, trademarks, service marks, etc. in this publication does not imply, even in the absence of a specific statement, that such names are exempt from the
relevant protective laws and regulations and therefore free for general use.
The publisher, the authors, and the editors are safe to assume that the advice and information in this book
are believed to be true and accurate at the date of publication. Neither the publisher nor the authors or the
editors give a warranty, expressed or implied, with respect to the material contained herein or for any
errors or omissions that may have been made. The publisher remains neutral with regard to jurisdictional
claims in published maps and institutional affiliations.

This Springer imprint is published by the registered company Springer Nature Switzerland AG
The registered company address is: Gewerbestrasse 11, 6330 Cham, Switzerland

Introduction

We are delighted to present to you the final product of an ever-evolving project to educate mental health clinicians, parents, and anyone else who is involved in the life of young people about the internet and social media. This book was originally presented as a symposium for the 2020 American Psychiatric Association Annual Meeting entitled "Teens, Screens and Social Connection: Problems and Solutions." At the time, we felt that updating clinicians on how children and adolescents use the internet was incredibly interesting and important. Little did we know that the COVID-19 Worldwide Pandemic would force us to present our symposium remotely from our homes instead of at a live conference in Philadelphia Pennsylvania.

As the quarantine progressed, we became accustomed to giving lectures, meeting and providing clinical care via online platforms. The internet and social media quickly became a lifeline for people of all ages to attend school, work and connect with others while being confined at home. We believe that the topic of this book, *Teens, Screens and Social Connection*, is even more timely and important now than it was back in early 2020. Life has changed immeasurably in the past several years, and it is important to understand where we have been and where we will be going in our digital lives.

The intersection of the digital world and mental health is an increasingly important topic and one that is especially pertinent to the pediatric and young adult population. Young people are spending an increasing amount of time on digital screen activities such as social media, texting, and online gaming. The vast majority of teens and pre-teens have access to computers and smartphones shifting social interaction away from face-to-face contact towards online communication. This provides both opportunities and challenges. A multitude of studies have described potential associations between mental illness and problematic internet use in youth. However, the digital world can also provide support, knowledge, and unique way of delivering mental health care to those in need.

This text will serve as a useful resource for mental health clinicians of different disciplines, as well as those who work with youth in other domains. It will provide concise yet comprehensive summary of this very timely and important topic. Not only will challenges be identified and described, but case studies and clinical pearls are provided that can be immediately applied to clinical practice.

In **Chap. 1: Diapers and Devices: The Effect of Screen Time on Early Childhood Psychological Developmental and Behaviors**, the author summarizes what we know (and do not know) about the effect of new media on the developing brain. Evaluation of a case study provides clinicians with a clear recommendation to give patients, families, or friends encountering the all-too-familiar scenario of excessive screen time in children.

The authors of **Chap. 2: Social Media and Screen Time in the Clinical Interview: What to Ask and What It Means?** prepare an extensive review of popular social media sites and how they function. This is invaluable knowledge for clinicians and will allow for a deeper understanding of how young patients are interacting online. They have included many examples of questions to use in the clinical interview, as well as ways of assessing for safety online in multiple domains.

A broad overview of social media as a unique entity is necessary in this volume. Clinicians need to have an understanding of modern technology through the eyes of their young patients. **Chap. 3: Introduction to the Virtual World: Pros and Cons of Social Media** provides the background and language which will prove helpful in understanding the following chapters. The topic of social media and social comparison is an especially interesting and relevant theme.

Chapter 4: Social Media's Influence on Identity Formation and Self-Expression briefly describes the main psychological theories of identity development and then applies this knowledge to the new phenomenon of the internet and social media. Important aspects of the social media experience are described, such as means of self-presentation, anonymity, privacy, and testing out different identities online. This chapter includes a special cultural addition exploring sex education and growing up LGBTQ+ in Latin America today.

Major Depressive Disorder is a disorder that commonly manifests during adolescence. **Chapter 5: Fear of Missing Out: Depression and the Internet** clarifies the connection between depression and social media through a review of the current evidence base. Both the direct and indirect factors between mood and social media use are discussed in this chapter, as well as ways to use this knowledge in therapeutic interactions.

A deep dive into a specialized type of bullying is taken in **Chap. 6: Social Media and Cyberbullying**. The explanations of the multiple types of cyberbullying are invaluable resource for clinicians. The difference between cyberbullying and bullying in real life is elucidated and put into the context of mental health. Helpful recommendations for clinicians and families are provided.

Chapter 7: Sexuality on the Internet: Identity Exploration, Cybersex, and Sexting sheds light on a common occurrence during adolescent development today. The potential negative outcomes of sexting are explored, as well as normative and positive effects. Clear recommendations on how to speak with youth are provided.

Chapter 8: Internet Gaming Disorder and Addictive Behaviors Online addresses the phenomenon of Internet Gaming Disorder (IGD), a proposed DSM diagnosis, which is seen increasingly often in clinical practice. Other addictive online behaviors, such as pornography and binge-watching are also discussed. Much needed guidance in treatment and prevention is offered.

Introduction vii

The positive aspects of the internet are often overlooked. **Chapter 9: Peer to Peer Support and the Strength of Online Communities** discusses the benefit of social media in the life of a teenager in today's society. The authors take a deeper look into how social media provides support, education, and a place for adolescents to feel included and empowered.

Given that the internet and social media are here to stay and play a large part in children's lives, **Chap. 10: Internet Safety: Family and Clinician Protection of Kids Online** provides a review of existing guidelines on internet safety and the role that parents and clinicians have in protecting children online.

The use of telepsychiatry has grown significantly during the COVID 19 pandemic so it was important to include **Chap. 11: Virtual Mental Health and Telepsychiatry: Opportunities and Challenges with Pediatric Patients** in this volume. This chapter discusses the benefits and challenges of virtual mental health in treating today's youth and their families. While telepsychiatry has allowed greater access to treatment for our patients, providers should also be mindful of when telepsychiatry is not an optimal treatment strategy.

Chapter 12: Lessons Learned from the COVID 19 Global Pandemic reviews how the COVID-19 pandemic has affected the mental health of children and adolescents. It details the multiple factors that have led to the increase in mental health crisis amongst youth. Even as COVID becomes a thing of the past, it is important to remember what we have learned during this difficult time in history.

We sincerely hope that you gain a better understanding and appreciation for the internet and social media from this volume. Modern technology is ubiquitous and here to stay, and it is impossible to predict the coming advancements of the future. We have found that the challenges associated with this new technology are not insurmountable, and that the positive factors are something that we could have only dreamed of as we were growing up. This evolution is bound to continue. It is important for all those who work with young people to continue to educate themselves in this arena. The internet is a rapidly moving target, but the benefits of understanding this world are unparalleled.

We want to take this opportunity to thank all our colleagues who contributed to this volume, especially the students, residents, and fellows who undertook such a Herculean task in addition to their already packed workloads and busy lives.

Alma Spaniardi
Janki Modi Avari

Contents

1 Diapers and Devices: The Effect of Screen Time on Early Childhood Psychological Development and Behavior ... 1
Hannah Simon

2 Social Media and Screen Time in the Clinical Interview: What to Ask and What It Means? ... 11
Ashvin Sood and Janki Modi Avari

3 Introduction to the Virtual World: Pros and Cons of Social Media ... 31
Jennifer Braddock, Sara Heide, and Alma Spaniardi

4 Social Media's Influence on Identity Formation and Self Expression ... 49
Maryann Tovar, Mineudis Rosillo, and Alma Spaniardi

5 Fear of Missing Out: Depression and the Internet ... 63
Sara Heide, Jennifer Braddock, and Alma Spaniardi

6 Social Media and Cyberbullying ... 79
Jenna Margolis and Dinara Amanbekova

7 Sexuality on the Internet: Identity Exploration, Cybersex and Sexting ... 103
Alice Caesar

8 Internet Gaming Disorder and Addictive Behaviors Online ... 113
Alex El Sehamy and Pantea Farahmand

9 Peer-to-Peer Support and the Strength of Online Communities ... 135
Alexandra Hamlyn and Pantea Farahmand

10 Internet Safety: Family and Clinician Protection of Kids Online ... 145
Renee C. Saenger and Anna H. Rosen

11 Virtual Mental Health and Telepsychiatry: Opportunities and Challenges with Pediatric Patients................................ 157
Jeffrey Anderson

12 Lessons Learned from the COVID-19 Global Pandemic............ 167
Rakin Hoq and Aaron Reliford

Index.. 179

Editors and Contributors

About the Editors

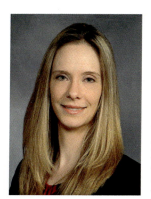

Alma Spaniardi, MD Service Chief of the Child and Adolescent Outpatient Department Payne Whitney Manhattan, Assistant Professor of Clinical Psychiatry Division of Child and Adolescent Psychiatry at Weill Cornell Medical College and Assistant Attending Psychiatrist at New York-Presbyterian Hospital. Dr. Spaniardi received her medical degree from Temple University School of Medicine and was a Phipps Resident in General Psychiatry at the Johns Hopkins Hospital Department of Psychiatry and Behavioral Sciences. She is trained in Child and Adolescent Psychiatry at the New York-Presbyterian Hospital's combined program of Columbia and Cornell Universities. She has extensive experience working in both inpatient and outpatient psychiatry as an attending psychiatrist on the adolescent inpatient unit at New York-Presbyterian Cornell Westchester and as an outpatient psychiatrist with the New York University Child Study Center. Dr. Spaniardi's clinical interests are quality improvement and the integration of psychiatry and pediatrics. She is an Editorial Board Member for the American College of Psychiatrists Resident's In-Training Examination (PRITE), regularly speaks at both national and international conferences and has contributed to several books on child psychiatry.

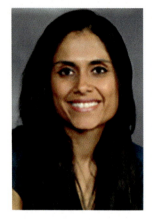

Janki Modi Avari, MD *Psychiatrist, child and adolescent psychiatrist, New York City Children's Center, Office of Mental Health-New York State.* Dr. Avari completed her adult psychiatry training at Mount Sinai Beth Israel Medical Center in New York City. She went on to do her child psychiatry training at the New York-Presbyterian Child and Adolescent training program, associated with Columbia University Medical Center and Weill Cornell Medical College. In her final year of fellowship, she was selected as a co-chief resident at Columbia University Medical Center. After graduation, Dr. Avari accepted a position at New York-Presbyterian Hospital and Weill Cornell Medical College, where she remained for 8 years. She is an assistant clinical professor of psychiatry and during her time at Weill Cornell, she was recipient of teaching and service awards. She currently works at New York State Office of Mental Health focusing on treating child and adolescents with treatment-resistant illness. Dr. Avari's areas of clinical interest are mood disorders and psychotic disorders in children and adolescents.

Contributors

Dinara Amanbekova, MD Department of Child and Adolescent Psychiatry, NYU Child Study Center, NYU Grossman School of Medicine, New York, NY, USA

Jeffrey Anderson, MD Department of Child and Adolescent Psychiatry, New York Presbyterian-Weill Cornell Medical College, New York, NY, USA

Janki Modi Avari, MD Office of Mental Health-New York City Children's Center, New York, NY, USA

Jennifer Braddock, BA New York University, New York, NY, USA

Alice Caesar, MD Department of Child and Adolescent Psychiatry, New York Presbyterian-Weill Cornell Medical College, New York, NY, USA

Alex El Sehamy, MD Department of Child and Adolescent Psychiatry, NYU Child Study Center, NYU Grossman School of Medicine, New York, NY, USA

Pantea Farahmand, MD Department of Child and Adolescent Psychiatry, NYU Child Study Center, NYU Grossman School of Medicine, New York, NY, USA

Diapers and Devices: The Effect of Screen Time on Early Childhood Psychological Development and Behavior

1

Hannah Simon

Case Study

You are asked to evaluate four-year-old Joe who, according to parents, is "addicted" to his electronic tablet. Joe spends upward of 3 h a day playing virtual games and watching youtube videos. Parents report that Joe will have tantrums and can become physically aggressive when parents attempt to set limits around tablet use. They also note that Joe will often stay up later than his bedtime to play on his tablet and appears more fatigued during the day. Parents first gave Joe a tablet when he was a toddler and downloaded educational apps to ensure that he was learning while engaging with his devices. They even read online in a parenting facebook group that some apps can help kids learn to read and get a head-start on kindergarten skills. Now Joe is struggling to meet academic milestones and lagging behind in reading, writing, and math in kindergarten. He is poorly socialized and struggles to make friends. What counseling would you offer to Joe's parents regarding screen time use?

Introduction

Early childhood is a period of enormous brain growth. During the first three years of life, experiences exert a profound influence on social, cognitive, and emotional development. While the innate processes that govern childhood development remain preserved across generations, the external environment surrounding our children has changed dramatically alongside the digital revolution of the last half-century. Unstructured play time and outdoor exploration have been replaced with screens,

---

H. Simon (✉)

Department of Child and Adolescent Psychiatry, New York Presbyterian-Weill Cornell Medical College, New York, NY, USA

e-mail: hcs9007@med.cornell.edu

© The Author(s), under exclusive license to Springer Nature Switzerland AG 2023

A. Spaniardi, J. M. Avari (eds.), *Teens, Screens, and Social Connection*,

https://doi.org/10.1007/978-3-031-24804-7_1

tablets, devices, and video games. Children are increasingly reliant on digital technology as both a means of entertainment as well as a tool for navigating their world. While parents have been counseled by pediatricians, teachers, and clinicians about the dangers of "too much screen time," the Covid-19 pandemic and realities of social distancing have increasingly propelled screens and digital technology to the forefront of our childrens' collective consciousness.

This chapter aims to examine current research on the effects of early screen time and digital media exposure on the cognitive, social, and emotional development in infants and young children. While there is a vast body of research focusing on television and video viewing in children, there is substantially less known about current media trends including more interactive platforms such as videogames and social apps. Much of the traditional research in this area focuses on school-age and adolescent children, with fewer studies primarily assessing outcomes in infants and toddlers. Given the enormous formative role of early childhood experience in establishing positive routines and habits as well as the degree of synaptic pruning that occurs during this time, it is imperative that we better understand and characterize how digital technology exposure influences developmental trajectories. Questions we will explore include the following: how does screen time usage vary across different demographic groups? Can excessive exposure to screen time have measurable and sustained effects on neurological, psychological, and behavioral development? Are there potential therapeutic interventions for digital technology? And how can parents, teachers, and clinicians apply present day research findings to guide recommendations regarding healthy use of digital technology in youngsters?

Epidemiological Review: Trends in Prevalence and Extent of Media Use Among Young Children

In 1999, the American Academy of Pediatricians (AAP) issued guidelines recommending parents to not expose television or screen entertainment to children under the age of two. These guidelines have since been modified to allow for videochatting (Facetime, Skype) in infants and toddlers as this practice is seen to promote social connectiveness among families [1]. These recommendations drew from years of research suggesting a lack of educational benefit, and in fact, potential adverse health and developmental impacts from media use in infants [2]. Despite these recommendations, media consumption among infants and toddlers has continued to skyrocket. Thirty years ago, children typically began to watch television starting at age four. In the most recent national survey conducted by Common Sense Media in 2020, children under the age of two average 49 min of screen time daily. Screen time usage increases with age, children from birth to age eight utilize about two and a half hours of screen media a day. Patterns of media use have shifted in young children to reflect technological trends: time spent in online video viewing (including *youtube* and social media videos) now surpasses television or DVD watching in children under eight years old. As devices have becomes more accessible and portable, children now spend increasingly more time engaging with media independently with less coparental monitoring [3].

While individual use varies widely, research indicates that socioeconomic differences correlate with amount and content of screen usage. In 2020, children in lower-income households spent an average of nearly two hours a day more with screen media than those in higher-income homes. Furthermore, children from lower-income households were also more likely to use technology for entertainment rather than educational purposes. Disparities in screen-time usage also continue to grow across racial divides; in 2020, Hispanic/Latinx and Black children spent on average one to two hours more time with screen media per day than White children do. These disparities may, in part, reflect different perceptions regarding the educational value of screen time in disadvantaged communities. In the most recent national survey, black parents and those from lower socioeconomic statuses were more likely to perceive educational benefits of screen time for their children relative to white and wealthier parents [2].

Research on Cognitive and Psychological Development in Young Children

For children under the age of two, research overwhelmingly shows a negative association between screen time and cognitive development. In a longitudinal study among infants, duration of screen-time exposure at 6 months was associated with lower cognitive development at 14 months as measured by Bayley Scales of Infant and Toddler Development [4]. Researchers from the Canadian Healthy Infant Longitudinal Developmental (CHILD) study, a naturalistic observation study of over 3,000 children in Canada, found a dose-dependent clinically significant relationship between increased screen-time exposure at ages three years of age and increased behavior problems at five years of age, as assessed by externalizing, internalizing, and total behavior problem scores on the Child Behavior Checklist. These effects persisted after controlling for associated factors including sleep duration, gender, socioeconomic status, parenting stress, and maternal depression [5]. Meta-analyses from additional studies have found negative associations between attentional symptoms and television viewing when young children were viewing more than two hours daily [6].

Research on Screen-Time Effect on Language Development

Research examining TV exposure has found significant associations between early life extensive screen exposure and language delays. In a study specifically looking at relationship between media exposure and language development in infants and toddlers (8–16 months), time spent viewing television and video content was inversely correlated with scores on validated communication inventories after adjusting for demographics and patient-child interactions [7]. These findings have been replicated in additional studies finding that children between the ages of 15 and 35 months frequently exposed to television had increased risk of language delays [8].

While there is compelling data linking screen time with lower language outcomes among young children, its associations with early brain development remains largely unknown. Researchers from the University of Cincinnati sought to elucidate neurobiological biomarkers in a landmark study comparing brain structures in preschool-age children with varying levels of screen usage. They found an association between increased screen-based media use and lower microstructural integrity of brain white matter tracts in brain regions involved in language and literacy skills in young children. These structural findings were supported by behavioral analyses, whereby high screen utilizers in the study scored lower on norm-referenced instruments testing reading and processing skills [9].

Screen-time Effect on Sleep

Later onset of sleep after evening media exposure has been documented in infants, and is especially pronounced in ethnic minority children [10]. This effect is thought to be due both to the stimulating nature of screen time as well as direct light exposure from devices interfering with melatonin production. In one study, infants exposed to screen media in the evening at six months of age had decreased 12-month night-time sleep duration [11]. Shorter sleep duration and disrupted quality of sleep in infants impacts crucial periods of early brain development and is correlated with delays in cognitive and motor development [12].

Limitations on Studies

It is important to note that there are limitations to the current research on screen-time exposures in young children. Determining causality between screen time and developmental outcomes is a fundamental challenge when very few randomized controlled trials exist in this area. Many studies do not account for other external variables linked to screen-time usage—socioeconomic status, parental level of education, stability of family structure, child baseline temperament—that strongly influence developmental outcomes. Studies traditionally have focused on viewing of television and videos with less research devoted to the newer digital technology including interactive and mobile media. It is unclear whether developmental outcomes from television research can be generalized to modern screen time as the way in which children interact with these technologies has changed drastically in the past twenty years. Likewise, the current body of research may not adequately capture media effects on infants and toddlers, as technology is now a more ubiquitous part of their lives. The impact of screen time on this younger cohort may be even more pronounced given their rapid and critical period of brain development. Furthermore, both the content and context of screen-time exposure are powerful determinants of psychological outcomes and may not be generalizable across studies. For example, while early exposure to adult-directed content tends to correlate with worse cognitive and behavioral outcomes, high-quality educational content does not confer these same risks.

Clinical Considerations

Experts propose a number of reasons of why excessive screen time is associated with negative developmental outcomes in young children. First and foremost, time spent engaging in digital technology is time lost to other critical activities. When a child is engrossed in their tablet, they are not playing make-believe, building a fort outside, helping their parent bake cookies, or attempting to make friends at a local park; all activities that research has shown are crucial for healthy neuropsychological development. Children that spend more time watching television or interfacing with digital media typically spend less time interacting with other family members or engaging in creative play. In households with heavy media use, children also spend significantly less time reading with parents. Simply having a television on in the background has been shown to distract from parent-child interaction and interfere with the quality of play [13].

The inappropriate adult-oriented content of screen time may also negatively influence psychological development in young children. While infants can begin to attend to screens beginning at around six months of age, they are not able to process and comprehend material presented on 2-dimensional screens until two years of age without the guidance of an adult. This may be due to the relative primitive nature of children's symbolic thinking to allow for transfer of knowledge from virtual to real platforms [14]. While infants may be able to mimic or imitate actions seen on screens, they are unable to consolidate new knowledge without an adult providing hands-on guidance. Interactions with caregivers are especially crucial for language development, as devices are not able to fully capture the human elements of reciprocal conversation- facial expressions, body language, and different social cues [15]. For these reasons, media exposure before the age of two serves little function in promoting acquisition of developmental milestones and, on the contrary, may actually impede neurocognitive and psychological growth.

Impact of Parental Screen Time

One of the most important predictors of problematic screen time usage in children is parental screen time. Studies find associations between high parental media usage and behavioral and emotional problems in young children. This effect may be mediated by lower quality and quantity of parent-child interactions when parents are engaged in their own mobile technology. Parent mobile technology use in the presence of the child has been shown to be associated with lower parental responsiveness, sensitivity, and attention to the child's needs [16].

There is also evidence that screen time may be used as a parenting intervention especially in children with baseline behavioral difficulties. Infants perceived by parents as having difficult temperaments generally have higher levels of TV exposure [17]. According to one study, children with social-emotional difficulties were more likely to be given mobile technology as a calming tool [18]. Parents often find the highly stimulating and distracting content of digital media can serve as an effective short-term solution for temper tantrums and behavioral outbursts. In the long term, however, using devices in this way can have a negative ripple effect both on childrens' ability to self-regulate their emotions and parents' reliance on devices as a parenting intervention. And as evidenced by longitudinal research studies, patterns of maladaptive media usage established in infancy often persist into adulthood.

Benefits of Screen Time and Technology

While in theory, screen time does not confer a significant benefit to infants and toddlers, in reality, media devices have become an essential part of our lives. Some experts propose that rather than implementing public health measures to curb the use of devices in children, we should instead focus our efforts toward innovating neuroscience-backed digital technology that promotes healthy psychological and cognitive development in youngsters. Many of these initiatives can draw from what scientists already know and understand about early childhood brain growth. For example, a substantial body of research has found educational age-appropriate television viewing (Sesame Street, Dora the Explorer) to positively influence prosocial behavior, vocabulary, and early school readiness in preschool-aged children and older [19]. Media that enables video-chatting or other forms of digital communication can provide social enrichment by connecting children to other friends or loved ones they may not otherwise interact with due to geographical barriers. Various studies have examined whether brain-training computer games can improve executive functioning such as task persistence, impulse control, emotion regulation, and flexible thinking. In children older than the age of six, one randomized controlled trial found significant improvements in ADHD symptoms six months after initiating a computerized working memory training program [20]. Another smaller study found benefits in literacy and math skills after providing low-income four-year-old children with IPod touches containing age-appropriate educational game software [21]. It is important to note that there are relatively few studies confirming therapeutic benefits of these novel technologies, and evidence is especially sparse as it pertains to infants and toddlers. As young children become increasingly digitized across the world, more research in this area is needed.

Recommendations

Let's return to the case study of Joe presented at the beginning of the chapter. Joe's parents introduced him to an electronic device as a toddler believing that it would provide him with educational benefits. Now, they struggle to set limits with screen time, and Joe's development has suffered as a result. How should you counsel this family?

1. **Time**: Start by asking parents how much time their child is spending on his device. In children between ages two under five, experts recommend limiting screen use to one hour per day of high-quality programs.

2. **Content**: Ask what the child is watching. Are the programs educational and enriching? Is the format more interactive or is he passively absorbing information presented on a screen? More interactive (including touch screen devices) and more educational content (including PBS or Sesame Street) confer greater benefits for learning and attention [22].

3. **Context**: ask when and how young children engage with devices. Do children watch screentime alone or with parents present? Are they handed a device to help diffuse a tantrum? To keep them quiet during meal times? At this age, it's important that parents or caregivers are actively coviewing content with children to help them better understand and learn from the media. Using screentime to curb tantrums can be a tempting quick fix, but over time this can impede children from learning how to self-regulate their emotions and can lead to problematic patterns of reinforcing negative behavior as a means of acquiring their highly addictive devices. Experts also recommend that young children avoid using screen time during designated times—before meals, during playtime, or bedtime. This ensures that screen time does not interfere with critical activities such as socializing, sleep, and creative exploration.

4. **Role of parental media use**: Encourage parents to examine how their own screen time usage can impact their young children's social and psychological development. In modeling healthy media use in the home, parents should consider when and how they engage in screen time, and limit background digital noise in the home whenever possible. While children below the age of 18 months may not be able to fully comprehend content presented on screens, they can certainly perceive the emotional value that parents place on their devices. Infants and toddlers may at times find themselves competing for parents' attention with the devices that rudely interrupt play time, and indeed, the research shows that excessive parental screen-time usage reduces both the quantity and quality of child-parent interactions.

5. **Balance**: Ensure adequate time is devoted to other critical developmental activities such as sleep, exercise, play time, and socialization. As discussed earlier, digital media impacts young child development both through the *direct* exposure to highly stimulating and often age-inappropriate content, as well as the indirect function of displacing other health-promoting activities.

6. Be sensitive to **socioeconomic barriers** that may enable excessive screen time use to go unchecked. It is important to recognize that in families with limited resources and without access to quality childcare, screen time can serve as a relatively inexpensive and accessible means of entertaining children and keeping problematic behaviors at bay. Expecting that parents completely eliminate all screen-time exposure in infants and toddlers may not be a realistic goal for many of these families. However, by providing parents with more practical guidelines guided by current research, clinicians can empower families to form a healthier relationship with technology.

Key Take-Home Points
- There are socioeconomic disparities in the prevalence and extent of screen time use.
- Excess exposure to screen time in young children is associated with delays in language, cognition, social development, and behavioral problems in school years.
- Children younger than 2 years require adult interaction to learn from screen media.
- Time interfacing with digital technology displaces activities critical for healthy development.
- Context and content of screen time matter.

Multiple Choice Questions
1. The majority of screen-time use in children under 8 years of age is spent on:
   A. Online videos
   B. TV/DVDs
   C. E-books
   D. Video Games
   E. Social media

Correct answer: A

2. How much screen time does the American Academy of Pediatrics (AAP) recommend daily for children under 24 months?
   A. None
   B. None, except when video-chatting with family
   C. <1 h daily
   D. <2 h daily
   E. >2 h daily of educational programming

Correct Answer: B

3. Which of the following is NOT an important consideration when counseling families on screen time?
   A. Content of screen time
   B. Context of when and how screen time is viewed
   C. Parental Media Use
   D. Size of device

Correct Answer: D

References

1. Chassiakos Y(L)R, Radesky J, Christakis D, Moreno MA, Cross C, Council on Communications and Media, Hill D, Ameenuddin N, Hutchinson J, Levine A, Boyd R, Mendelson R, Swanson WS. Children and adolescents and digital media. Pediatrics. 2016;138(5):e20162593. https://doi.org/10.1542/peds.2016-2593.
2. Brown A. Council on communications and media; media use by children younger than 2 years. Pediatrics. 2011;128(5):1040–5. https://doi.org/10.1542/peds.2011-1753.
3. Rideout V, Robb MB. The Common Sense census: media use by kids age zero to eight, 2020. San Francisco, CA: Common Sense Media; 2020.

1 Diapers and Devices: The Effect of Screen Time on Early Childhood Psychological... 9

4. Tomopoulos S, Dreyer BP, Berkule S, Fierman AH, Brockmeyer C, Mendelsohn AL. Infant media exposure and toddler development. Arch Pediatr Adolesc Med. 2010;164(12):1105–11. https://doi.org/10.1001/archpediatrics.2010.235.
5. Tamana SK, Ezeugwu V, Chikuma J, Lefebvre DL, Azad MB, Moraes TJ, et al. Screen-time is associated with inattention problems in preschoolers: results from the CHILD birth cohort study. PLoS One. 2019;14(4):e0213995. https://doi.org/10.1371/journal.pone.0213995.
6. Duch H, Fisher EM, Ensari I, Harrington A. Screen time use in children under 3 years old: a systematic review of correlates. Int J Behav Nutr Phys Act. 2013;10:102. https://doi.org/10.1186/1479-5868-10-102.
7. Zimmerman FJ, Christakis DA, Andrew N. Meltzoff associations between media viewing and language development in children under age 2 years. J Pediatr. 2007;151(4):364–8. https://doi.org/10.1016/j.jpeds.2007.04.071.
8. Chonchaiya W, Pruksananonda C. Television viewing associates with delayed language development. Acta Paediatr. 2008;97(7):977–82.
9. Hutton JS, Dudley J, Horowitz-Kraus T, DeWitt T, Holland SK. Associations between screen-based media use and brain white matter integrity in preschool-aged children. JAMA Pediatr. 2020;174(1):e193869. https://doi.org/10.1001/jamapediatrics.2019.3869.
10. Miller EB, Canfield CF, Wippick H, Shaw DS, Morris PA, Mendelsohn AL. Predictors of television at bedtime and associations with toddler sleep and behavior in a medicaid-eligible, racial/ethnic minority sample. Infant Behav Dev. 2022;6:101707.
11. Vijakkhana N, Wilaisakditipakorn T, Ruedeekhajorn K, Pruksananonda C, Chonchaiya W. Evening media exposure reduces night-time sleep. Acta Paediatr. 2015;104:306–12. https://doi.org/10.1111/apa.12904.
12. Tham EK, Schneider N, Broekman BF. Infant sleep and its relation with cognition and growth: a narrative review. Nat Sci Sleep. 2017;9:135–49. https://doi.org/10.2147/NSS.S125992.
13. Anderson DR, Subrahmanyam K, On Behalf of the Cognitive Impacts of Digital Media Workgroup. Digital screen media and cognitive development. Pediatrics. 2017;140(Supplement_2):S57–61. https://doi.org/10.1542/peds.2016-1758C.
14. Courage ML, Howe ML. To watch or not to watch: infants and toddlers in a brave new electronic world. Dev Rev. 2010;30:101–15.
15. https://healthmatters.nyp.org/what-does-too-much-screen-time-do-to-childrens-brains/
16. Poulain T, Ludwig J, Hiemisch A, Hilbert A, Kiess W. Media use of mothers, media use of children, and parent-child interaction are related to behavioral difficulties and strengths of children. Int J Environ Res Public Health. 2019;16(23):4651. https://doi.org/10.3390/ijerph16234651.
17. Thompson AL, Adair LS, Bentley ME. Maternal characteristics and perception of temperament associated with infant TV exposure. Pediatrics. 2013;131(2):e390–7. https://doi.org/10.1542/peds.2012-1224.
18. Radesky JS, Peacock-Chambers E, Zuckerman B, et al. Use of mobile technology to calm upset children: associations with social-emotional development. JAMA Pediatr. 2016;170(4):397–9.
19. Fisch SM. Children's learning from educational television: "Sesame Street" and beyond. Mahwah, NJ: Lawrence Erlbaum; 2004.
20. Bigorra A, Garolera M, Guijarro S, Hervás A. Long-term far-transfer effects of working memory training in children with ADHD: a randomized controlled trial. Eur Child Adolesc Psychiatry. 2016;25(8):853–67. https://doi.org/10.1007/s00787-015-0804-3. Epub 2015 Dec 15.
21. Griffith SF, Hanson KG, Rolon-Arroyo B, Arnold DH. Promoting early achievement in low-income preschoolers in the United States with educational apps. J Children Media. 2019;13(3):328–44. https://doi.org/10.1080/17482798.2019.1613246.
22. Kirkorian HL, Choi K, Pempek TA. Toddlers' word learning from contingent and noncontingent video on touch screens. Child Dev. 2016;87(2):405–13.

Social Media and Screen Time in the Clinical Interview: What to Ask and What It Means?

2

Ashvin Sood and Janki Modi Avari

Introduction

Children and teenagers live in a digital age. Phones, tablets, laptops, desktops, watches, and other devices are ubiquitous in both the home environment and the school environment. Whether it is getting a snapchat notification at breakfast or learning a new Tiktok dance after school, youth's exposure to digital media, whether it is a social media platform or an entertainment medium, is a phenomenon that occurs in a majority of households. Yet, what is the landscape in which digital content presents itself to youth and how do we screen and assess the amount of time as well as type of content our patients' consume? To answer these questions, we need to first understand the backdrop of digital media and the prevalent trends of how children and teenagers participate in the virtual landscape.

Over the past two decades, children under the age of 18 have dramatically increased their time viewing screens: 12th graders' internet use during leisure time doubled between 2006 and 2016 (from about 1 h a day to about 2 h a day.) In that same time, 8th graders' internet time increased by 68% and 10th graders' internet time increased by 75% [1]. In 2015, Common Sense Media, a nonprofit organization that examines children and teen media use, noted that 57% of teenagers spend more than 4 h per day with screen media [2]. However, these numbers appear outdated when examining screen media time and use during the COVID-19 pandemic. In the STROBE (Strengthening the Reporting of Observational Studies in Epidemiology) study, 5,412 adolescents between the ages of 12 to 13 were asked to assess their screen time use prior to the pandemic and postpandemic, with average

---

A. Sood (✉)
SSM Health Treffert Studios, Fond Du Lac, Wisconsin, USA

J. M. Avari
Office of Mental Health-New York City Children's Center, New York, NY, USA

© The Author(s), under exclusive license to Springer Nature Switzerland AG 2023
A. Spaniardi, J. M. Avari (eds.), *Teens, Screens, and Social Connection*,
https://doi.org/10.1007/978-3-031-24804-7_2

screen time increasing from 3.8 h to 7.7 h; [3] 8–12-year olds are not far behind, averaging 4 h and 44 min of screen media a day [4]. Parental reports of teen screen time have also indicated significant changes as well. In a poll conducted by Morning Consult, 32% of parents believed their teens had used electronic devices daily for more than 4 hours before the COVID-19 pandemic. In contrast, as of June 2020, 62% of parents from the same sample population believed their teens had used electronic devices daily for more than 4 h [5].

If screen time use is increasing, on what device are children and teenagers consuming digital content? Per Pew research, 95% of U.S. teenagers have access to a smartphone, a two-fold increase over the 41% teen smartphone ownership reported in 2012 [6]. Children also follow a similar trend, with 53% of children 11 and younger owning a smartphone. As smart phone use has increased, other modalities have decreased in response. The number of teenagers watching television on a television set has decreased from 64% to 50% during the period 2015–2019, while the number of teenagers watching television on a smartphone has increased from 6% to 20% [4]. Tablet computers appear to follow a rising trend of use, albeit smaller, in the younger age groups. For example, when asked about the appropriate age for their child to have or own their own tablet, 65% of parents agreed that their child owning a tablet before the age of 12 was acceptable, while only 22% of parents believed it was acceptable to own a smartphone before the age of 12 [7].

Given the increase in screen time, what are children and teenagers consuming digitally? Per Common Sense Census in 2019, which analyzed the results of 1600 8–18-year olds about their relationship with screen media, tween screen time was dominated by television and video use (53%), gaming (31%), browsing websites (5%), and social media (4%.) Similarly, teens also consumed television and videos primarily (39%) and followed by gaming (22%). However, social media use rose significantly to 16% among teens compared to their younger counterparts [4]. Per the GlobalWebIndex Report of 2018, teens and young adults between the ages of 16–24 averaged 3 h on social media daily. Rates of multiple daily engagements in social media have also risen dramatically as well, rising from 38% in 2012 to 70% in 2018, including 16% who say they use it "almost constantly [8]."

Social media is vast and covers numerous platforms. With over 4.48 billion active social media users globally, giants such as Facebook, Instagram, Snapchat, and Twitter have dominated the digital playground [9]. In 2015, 71% of teens aged 13–17 reported they used Facebook as their primary social media platform, followed by Instagram (52%), Snapchat (41%), and Twitter (31% [6].) However, digital trends are altered at remarkably fast speeds. Pipler Sandler Investment Research surveyed 9,800 teens in the fall of 2020, asking which social media sites were most popular. Surprisingly, Snapchat had become the most favored social platform (34%), followed by the new social media platform Tiktok (29%), then instagram (25%), with Facebook falling last (2%.) Highest engagement or actual reported use tells a slightly different story, with Instagram used most (84%), followed by Snapchat (80%), then Tiktok (69% [10].)

This chapter will focus on educating the clinician on how to screen children and teen screen time and social media use. It will not focus on content outside of social media, that of which may include digital entertainment, such as netflix or youtube, or video game consumption. Those areas of digital entertainment are vast and require their own separate chapters. The first part of this chapter will discuss what aspects clinicians are looking for in the clinical interview that would raise concern. The second part of this chapter will explore how clinicians can ask questions regarding screen time and social media and how confidentiality should be approached.

Screening Strategies

Screen Time: The Overarching Areas of Emphasis and Interests are When, Where, and How Much?

Initially, the American Academy of Pediatrics originally suggested that there should be discouragement of media use under the age of 2, with specific parameters limiting time with screens for different age groups [11]. However, as the virtual playground has evolved, more nuanced recommendations have arrived on advising families on media use, specifically based on where and when screen time is occurring. But when does screen time occur and in what settings?

Screen time appears to peak in the late afternoon and into the evenings for the majority of children and teenagers, with a second smaller peak occurring in the morning for younger children. Regarding weekdays and weekend use, all family members tend to use electronics more comparatively on weekends than weekdays, with older children and teenagers having more screen time than their younger counterparts [12]. To further illustrate this trend, a sample of 1,448 children aged 7 and below and 1,517 children aged 7–10 were followed by their parents to assess their change in screen time. Parents noted that while their children watched 2 hours of TV on a weekday, that number rose approximately by 75% and 74%, respectively, on the weekend [13].

Regarding times of day, evening and night time screen use appear to be the most common for teenagers. Seventy five percent of American children and adolescents report the presence of at least 1 screen media device in their bedroom, with roughly 60% reporting regular use of these devices during the hour before bedtime [14]. Adolescent night social media use was typically driven by concerns over negative consequences for real-world relationships if they disconnected. These concerns were related to peer-exclusion and fear of violating social norms around online availability [15]. The consequences of screen time use at night are well documented. A meta-analysis of 20 studies examined 125,000 youth, and results indicated that bedtime media usage is associated with negative consequences on sleep. Insufficient sleep duration, poor sleep quality, and excessive daytime sleepiness were all such outcomes. The mere presence of a portable screen-based media device in the bedroom has adverse associations with sleep outcomes [16].School also plays a part in smartphone use. While recent data is still pending, Pew Research Center's Internet and American Life Project from 2009 noted that 77% of teenagers bring their phone to school [17]. This number has certainly risen over the past decade.

Social Media Applications

There are numerous social media applications that can be accessed by phone, tablet, computer, and other smart devices with certain tech monoliths ruling the digital arena. Facebook (now known as "Meta") continues to have the most active users with over 2.895 billion users globally in 2021, followed by Youtube (2.291 billion users), WhatsApp (2 billion users), and Instagram (1.386 billion [18]). However, attention has shifted to other platforms, namely, Tiktok and Snapchat, as these platforms appear to be targeting younger audiences and growing in popularity. Currently, Tiktok has 732 million active users globally, with 47.4% of Tiktok's user base in the United States aged between 10 and 29 years old [19]. Snapchat has 293 million users globally, with 48% of their user base in the United States aged between 15 and 25 years old [20]. Though active in the teen community, only 39% of Instagram's user base falls under the 13–24 age range [21]. Per Piper Sandler, an investment firm that takes stock of teen use and social media, Snapchat still remains the main social media application for teens, followed by Tiktok and Instagram [22]. For this chapter, we will go over how Tiktok, Snapchat, and Instagram work, and what parts of these applications clinicians should be aware of.

Tiktok is a short-form video sharing application that allows users to upload 0–180 s video clips. Each video clip can be linked with audio or associated sounds such as voice recordings, music, and dialogue. If a user is not creating videos themselves, they have the option to swipe through other users' videos in a relatively quick manner. Tiktok's digital layout offers five different choices that a user can select, including a home page, discover page, creation page, an inbox page, and personal page. Briefly, the home page features videos from creators that the user is actively following (such as a celebrity or a friend that often creates video content) or a "For You" page, which shows videos that Tiktok believes the user would enjoy. For the latter, Tiktok's algorithm of picking those videos for users is based on numerous criteria, including accounts users follow, comments users have posted, themes behind videos that users watch (sports, video gaming, etc.), and most importantly, how long users have remained on a video (watching portions of a video vs. the entirety of the video.) On the discover page, users see the latest trending sounds or hashtags that are gaining popularity, and are encouraged to create content on the creation page with similar favorable attributes. The inbox page allows users to see how many individuals are actively liking, commenting, and sharing their videos. Finally, the personal page shows users their videos that they have personally uploaded, the amount of "likes" in total that their videos have received, the amount of followers they have, and how many accounts the user is following. Tiktok also has a messaging service in which users can direct message each other (also known as "DM" [23, 24].)

Snapchat is a social media application that prides itself on a simple concept: any picture or video that a user sends is only available to the recipient for a short time before it becomes inaccessible. Initially focused on person-to-person sharing, Snapchat has expanded to sending short videos, live video chatting, direct messaging, creating caricature-like bitmoji avatars, and sharing a chronological

"Story" that's broadcasted to all followers. When opening the Snapchat application, users are greeted to their phone's camera interface. On the bottom of the screen, users will see a capture button, which they can either press (or hold) to take pictures and videos for up to 10 s long. After taking the "snap," users can write texts, add stickers, or color on to their photos or videos, and then choose to either upload it to their story page where all users can see their content or directly message other users privately. If users wish to save their own photos or videos they have sent to others, they can save their media on the memory page. However, users are notified if others try to save their photos via taking a screenshot. Similar to Tiktok, Snapchat also has a discover page, where popular stories are posted by media outlets that expire after 24 h. One other aspect of Snapchat is the Snap map, a tool in which users can see the exact location of where people sent their latest snaps. This is an optional feature and users can put their profile in "ghost mode" for which no other user can see their location [25–27].

Launching in 2010, Instagram is the oldest of the 3 most consumed social media sites among teenagers. Similar to Facebook (which serves as owner now), Instagram allows users to follow other users' content, generating a homepage with information known as a "feed " on the user's home page. The feed is filled with posts created by individuals, groups, and companies for which the user follows. Instagram also has an explore page (similar to Tiktok's discover page) that hosts pictures and videos for which the user can interact with, leading to the application making similar recommendations in the future. At the top of the home page, users will see the "story" section, where other users have posted short video clips of the day's events for which a population (selected or general) can view. Similar to SnapChat, these stories expire after 24 hours unless saved by the user who posted the story. Above the story section is a small icon linked to a DM service in which users can connect with each other (again, similar to Tiktok and Snapchat.) Other pages on the application include a shop page, where users can buy various products sold through the platform as well as a profile icon, where users can see how many followers they have or who they are following. As Instagram has had to adapt to compete with other social media applications, they have also jumped into the digital video market. Instagram Reels is similar to Tiktok, and allows users to post short videos with selected audio that other users can view. Instagram also allows for longer videos (several minutes to an hour) to be posted under the category of IGTV or Instagram television [28–30].

Reasons for Teenage Use of Social Media

In the digital age where over 85% of teenagers are on social media, clinicians may be scratching their heads to ask what's the purpose behind their interest with these platforms [31]. A meta-analytic review of studies of the reasons behind Facebook addiction, for example, found that the major motivations to use facebook included relationship maintenance, entertainment, companionship, and simply "passing time [32]." Reasons are vast, but the leading category of interest appears to fall under the category of connection and peer support. A 2019 survey consisting of

6,247 respondents aged 13–29 reported that 84% of young individuals use social media for purpose of communicating with friends [33]. Fifty seven percent of teens aged 13–17 have made a new friend online, and 62% of teens share their social media username when they meet someone for the first time. Twenty-three percent of teens indicate that they spend time with friends on social media every day [34]. Regarding actual perceived support, gender differences exist, where 73% of girls endorse receiving emotional support from peers compared to 63% of boys. Teens also highlight that social media has made it easier to communicate with family and friends, with benefits including increased self-esteem and increased opportunities of self-disclosure [35]. Other aspects of connection stem from what teens post on social media sites. Disclosure of accomplishments, followed by family-related events and then emotional feelings tended to be highly popular on social media sites such as Instagram [6].

Entertainment serves as a primary reward from social media use. In the UK, users of the social media site TikTok highlighted categories such as comedy, dancing, watching others lip sync songs, and animals as main reasons behind application use [36]. While Youtube continues to remain the top contender for entertainment purposes through streaming online video content, 36–40% of parents with children aged 13–17 report that Instagram and Tiktok are the most popular entertainment applications in their household [37]. Entertainment entities such as HBO, Netflix, Amazon, and even children's television such as Cartoon Network and Nickelodeon have active, thriving social media accounts that boast millions of followers.

Education, prior to the pandemic, had less of a following compared to connection and entertainment. Per Common Sense Media, many teens agree that social media helps them to be more aware of current events, but there was a drop in the percent who "strongly agree" with that statement, from 26 percent in 2012 to 18 percent in 2018 [38]. However, one year into the pandemic, Common Sense Media released new data, highlighting that 8 in 10 youth (85%) have looked for health information online, with "depression," "stress," and "anxiety" among the top searches, with social media serving as a primary source of information [39]. Self-expression through content creation serves as a pillar, albeit smaller, when it comes to uses behind social media. In 2018, 37 percent of teens said creative posting, through text messages or video, was "somewhat" important, with girls highlighting this purpose as "very important" compared to boys [38]. However, like education, self-expression has increased significantly with the rising popularity of short-uploaded videos via snapchat, Tiktok, and Instagram's Reels.

Gender Differences and Social Media

Significant evidence indicates that adolescent girls and gender minority youth are more emotionally invested in social media than their cisgender male youth [40]. Both populations have reported spending higher average daily hours on social media and higher frequency of checking social media [41]. Additionally, earlier age of onset of social media use has correlated with worse emotional well-being scores in females compared to males [42]. Theories suggest that adolescent females, in pre-pubertal and pubertal years, are often engaged in upward social comparison, or the ability to compare oneself to someone who is perceived as better than they are [43]. When teens view peer or celebrity profiles who post photos or text that highlight accomplishments (whether based on physical beauty, social status, wealth, or relationship status), values of self-esteem and self-evaluation can plummit [44].

Detrimental Effects of Social Media

A teenager's mental health is connected to their digital world, depending on the state of the teenager's emotional well-being. In 2018, Common Sense Media conducted a survey for teenagers asking questions relating to happiness, depression, loneliness, confidence, self-esteem, and parental relations. Questions such as "I am happy with my life" and "I often feel sad or depressed" were asked and based on the teenager's response, a social emotional well-being (SEWB) score was calculated. The higher the score, the higher the social emotional well-being of the teenager. Results indicated that those who had "low" SEWB scores tended to find social media significantly more important and impactful to their day-to-day lives. Teenagers with low SEWB scores compared to teenagers with high SEWB scores reported feeling left out or excluded when using social media (70% vs. 29%), more likely to delete their social media posts, because they got too few "likes" (43% vs. 11%), felt bad about themselves if no one commented on or liked their post (43% vs. 11%) and were more likely to have been cyberbullied (35% vs. 5% [38].)

Self-esteem and worth also play a part in how a teenager interacts with social media. Self-esteem levels and emotional investment in social media are negatively correlated, highlighting that those who value their digital connection are more at risk for requiring external validation through likes, views, and amount of followers [45, 46]. Poor sleep also correlates with social media use. It is well known that adolescents who have access to screens late at night have poorer quality of sleep, shorter durations of sleep, and difficulty in falling asleep compared to their nonscreen time counterparts [47, 48]. However, night-time-specific social media use, with constant notifications, access to direct messaging other peers, and the fear of missing out on social activities, is now linked to worsening sleep quality among adolescents [49]. In return, poor quality of sleep leads to issues with executive function, motor control (potentially leading to motor vehicle accidents when sleepy teenagers drive to school), and difficulty with declarative and working memory [49–52].

Remaining on topic regarding vulnerable youth, teenagers with pre-existing psychiatric illnesses are also at risk of worsening their mental health while on social media. Research conducted in Canada highlighted that teenagers with depression were more vulnerable to experiencing negative experiences (loneliness, etc.) on social media sites such as Facebook [53]. Anxious adolescents tend to use social media more, and teenagers who utilized more hours of social media with pre-existing anxiety disorders tended to worsen their anxiety [54, 55]. Prevalence of eating disorders has also increased as social media use has risen among adolescents

[56]. Teenagers often find themselves comparing their body shape and size to other users, subscribing to dieting trends, or following models and celebrities that pride themselves on their physique. Numerous studies have highlighted how photo-based media sites such as Instagram have served as risk factors for developing poor body image, increased perception of fatness, and greater disordered eating attitudes, particularly among adolescent females [57]. Those who have problematic social networking use, such as high degree of emotional investment in social media, are also more likely to develop disordered eating symptoms [58].

Signs of Youth at Risk

Engaging in social media use by teenagers isn't necessarily a bad thing. Connection, support, education, entertainment, and self-expression are important for adolescent growth and maturation. However, certain behaviors and experiences can put teens at risk for demoralization, sexual and emotional abuse, self-harm, and suicidality. These experiences should be screened and assessed when discussing an adolescent's activity on social media.

Cyberbullying is a well-documented and prevalent phenomenon plaguing teenagers and causing significant emotional distress. In a systematic review conducted in 2021, cyberbullying victimization and perpetration among those under the age of 18 globally ranged were 14.6–52.2% and 6.3–32%, respectively [59]. There are multiple different forms of cyberbullying including verbal violence, group violence, visual violence, impersonating and account forgery, sexual harassment, and cyberstalking (Table 2.1) [60]. Individuals who endure cyberbullying are more likely to endorse symptoms of anxiety, depression, and suicidal ideation compared to non-victimized peers [61, 62]. Different social media sites such as Instagram, Snapchat, and Tiktok are notoriously connected to acts of cyberbullying. In a 2017 survey conducted by Ditch the Label, a nonprofit antibullying group, more than 1 in 5 12–20-year olds experience bullying specifically on Instagram [63]. Hate pages, a mixture of group violence and account forgery, are an example of cyberbullying,

Table 2.1 Outlined here are the different types of cyberbullying

Term	Definition
Verbal violence	Behavior of offensive responses, insults, mocking, threats, slander, and harassment targeted at victim 49
Group violence	Preventing others from joining certain groups or isolating others, forcing others to leave the group
Visual violence	Releasing and sharing embarrassing and private photos and information without the owner's consent
Impersonating and account forgery	Identity theft, stealing passwords, violating accounts, and the creation of fake accounts to fraudulently present behavior of others
Sexual harassment	Unwelcomed sexual conduct that the victim does not consent to on a digital media platform
Cyberstalking	Harassing or stalking a victim online via direct messaging or other forms of electronic communication

where a page is created to insult and demean a victim while encouraging others to post similar content about the victim [64].Bullying also occurs through SnapChat and Tiktok as well. In 2021, SnapChat had to suspend two particular applications that allowed users to send anonymous messages to other users after a teenager committed suicide, invoking an ensuing lawsuit by the parent of the teenager. The parent's reason for the lawsuit stemmed from the numerous hateful and offensive messages that their teenager received from anonymous sources days prior to his suicide completion [65]. Tiktok has also faced its fair share of criticism, with users who post videos and then face an onslaught of racial, homophobic, and body shaming commentary by other users [66].

Sexual exploitation via digital media is an unfortunate reality for children and teenagers. Nearly 1 in 7 children aged 9–12 shared their own nude photos in 2020, almost tripling the number from just one year earlier [67]. The number of sexual texts ("sexts") children and teens have attempted to send (including girls as young as 6) has risen over 183% during the pandemic [68]. Perception of sharing sexually explicit images of oneself is also shifting. Recently, 40% of teenagers agreed that "it's normal for people my age to share nudes with each other" [69]. Additionally, nearly 40% of children have either received and/or sent a "sext" by the age of 13 [69]. Social media applications serve as a medium for nude photos ("nudes") as well. Articles, such as "How to Sext on Snapchat Like a Pro," highlight ways in which users can send sexually explicit content to each other [70]. Instagram has also created a "vanish mode," a feature in which users can have their messages deleted after a chat box is closed. Vanish mode has been characterized by many users as manner in which sexually explicit images can be sent between users without the fear of future exploitation [71]. However, consequences of nude pictures being released into the online universe are well known. Adolescent teenagers, primarily girls, have suffered from their intimate photos being shared with peer groups without their consent [72]. Per the Federal Bureau of Investigations (FBI), online sexual exploitation comes in many forms, with perpetrators coercing victims into providing sexually explicit images or videos of themselves, often in compliance with the offender(s) threats to post the images publicly or send the images to victims' friends and family [73]. Through direct messaging and introducing themselves or "liking" posts gaining a child or adolescent's attention via social media platforms, sexual offenders often target vulnerable youth by gaining their trust through validation and affirmation. Once a connection is created, coercion and manipulation by a sexual offender can lead to the child or adolescent sending sexually graphic texts and photos, which then the sexual offender can use to extort their victims into dangerous behaviors (sexual favors, crime, etc.)

As discussed earlier, teenagers aim to connect with their peers regarding their vulnerable feelings through various forms of communication on social media. However, the content of messages can also place recipients of those messages in precarious positions, primarily when those messages relate to self-harm and suicide. Posts relating to nonsuicidal self-injurious behavior (NSSIB) have dramatically increased. For instance, teens posted between 58,000 and 68,000 images with hashtags (markers that are picked up by social media algorithms to send to users who also use similar markers in their posts) related to some form of self-injury in February of 2018. By December of 2018, that figure has increased to over 112,000 images with notable hashtags including #selfharm, #hatemyself, and #selfharmawareness [74]. Clinicians have also reported similar findings when interviewing teens. A study surveying 94 licensed clinicians found that 30.9% reported at least some of their clients who self-injured had utilized the internet to share NSSIB images with other peers [75]. The dangers of viewing NSSIB online stem from contagion, or the spreading of ideas and information that can be acted on by parties who may have not been actively participating in NSSIB. Individuals with a history of NSSIB who are actively exposed to NSSIB-related content may have cravings to enact self-injury [76]. Gender is also an important factor to consider.

Screening

As highlighted, understanding how social media works, what social media applications are most commonly used, the purpose behind social media, and the detrimental effects of social media are incredibly important for clinicians. During the psychiatric interview, a child or teen may seem to have a straightforward day-to-day routine, but their digital world can be incredibly complex. Below are questions in which clinicians can use to determine if a child or teenager is suffering from, or at risk for, negative consequences of social media use. Questions for both parents and the child/teenager are included in Table 2.2 [77].

Table 2.2 Questions parents and clinicians should use to better understand social media usage

Screen time and sleep	• What time of the day do you use your smartphone the most? • If you use it at night, do you use it in your bedroom? • If so, how late would you say you stay up using your smartphone? • How long can you go without checking your phone while you are in bed? • Have your parents ever had to take your smartphone away, because you were staying up too late? • What time do you have to wake up for school?
Smartphone use in school	• How often do you check your smartphone at school? • Are your peers using their smartphones in school? If so, what are they using it for? • Does your school allow you to use your smartphone in class? • If so, are there times when you are not allowed to use it? • Have you ever gotten into trouble for using your phone?
Social media application preference	• Do you use social media such as Instagram, Snapchat, Tiktok, etc.? • If so, is there one that you use more than others? • What do you use it for? Some examples could include talking with friends, scrolling through posts, or creating content. Are any of those important to you?

Table 2.2 (continued)

If child/teen uses Tiktok	• Do you scroll through videos and/or do you create content? • If you create content, what would a video look like? • Could you show me one of your videos? • If you don't create content, what pops up on your For You Page? • To get a better understanding of who you are, could I see your For You Page? • How many followers do you have? • Are having a lot of followers important to you? • Do you use the direct messaging feature on Tiktok? If so, do you send DMs to anyone in particular? • Have you ever compared yourself to individuals on Tiktok? If so, how did you feel afterward?
If child/teen uses Snapchat	• Do you send snaps? If so, to whom do you send the most snaps to? Are they mostly videos or pictures? • Are there snap groups you are a part of? • Do you follow anyone's story? Is there one that you follow more than others? • Are you on SnapMap? If so, who can see your location? • Do you use ghost mode? • Do you use direct messaging (DM) on Snapchat? • Are there any snaps you have saved? May I see what snap memories you have saved? • Do you ever use filters to change your appearance? How did they change your appearance? • Have you ever compared yourself to individuals on snapchat? If so, how did you feel afterward? • Are there any Snaps you sent that you regret?
If child/teen uses Instagram	• Who or what do you follow on Instagram? • Is there a theme (like makeup, sports, celebrities, etc.) in the accounts you follow? • What topics would I find on your explore page? • Do you use direct messaging (DM) on Instagram? • Do you spend time looking at Instagram Reels? What about Instagram TV (IGTV)? • Whose stories do you follow on Instagram? • Do you buy anything on the shop page for Instagram? • Have you ever compared yourself to individuals on Instagram? If so, how did you feel afterward?
Cyberbullying	• Have your friends, peers, or strangers commented on your posts in a negative manner? • Have individuals sent you aggressive or mean direct messages? • Have you ever been the subject of a group text where others say mean things about you? • Has there been a time where you were kicked out of an online group? • Have you ever come across a hate page on Instagram? If so, what did you think about it? • Have you ever been the subject of a hate page? • Have others body shamed you on social media? • Has anyone ever shared sensitive and private information about you (such as your sexuality, sexual history, drug use, etc.) to others without your consent?

(continued)

Table 2.2 (continued)

Sexually explicit information	• Do your friends sext or send nudes on snapchat, Instagram, or Tiktok? If so, how do you feel about that? • Have you ever received nude photos from another user on snapchat or another form of social media / text? Has this ever been against your consent? • Have you ever sent a nude photo of yourself, or parts of your body, to another individual on snapchat or another form of social media/text? • Have others pressured you into sending a nude photo? • If they have, did they threaten you by withholding affection or sharing sensitive information about you with others? • Do you go online to start romantic or sexual relationships? Did you meet these people in person?
Self-harming behavior	• Have you come across posts where people talk about self-harm? • Are there videos you have seen on Tiktok, Snapchat, or Instagram Reels where individuals have self-harmed? Are these common themes on your For You Page (Tiktok) and Explore page (Instagram)? • Has anyone disclosed to you that they self-harmed through direct message? What has been your response? • Do images of self-harm affect you in any particular way? • Have you sent direct messages to friends about feeling like you want to self-harm? How have they reacted? • Do you notice that you want to self-harm more when you come across self-harm videos?
Parental Report	• How many hours is your child on their phone a day? • Are there rules regarding screen time? And if so, are they enforced similarly on weekdays and weekends? • Do they sleep with their phone in their room? • Are there rules about phone use at night before bedtime? • Does your child/teenager stay up past their bedtime on their phone? • If phone use is restricted/taken away, how does your child react? • Has your child ever gotten into trouble regarding their phone use at school? • What kind of screen time was allowed during the early years? How did you supervise this? • What are your (parents) phone habits? Are there phone rules that are followed by everyone in the household? • Regarding social media, are you aware of what social media applications your teenager is on? If so, which one seems to be the most predominantly used? • Does your child or teen have a public profile or do they have a private profile on Instagram, Snapchat, or Tiktok? • Are you aware of any cyberbullying that your child or teenager participates in or is a victim of? • Are you aware of any sexually explicit activities that your child or teen may be participating in social media? • Do you have any privacy control measures or digital applications that assist in monitoring what your child participates in?

Confidentiality and Specific Considerations

Children and teenagers sharing aspects of their digital presence can be an incredibly vulnerable experience. Their digital interactions and experiences highlight parts of their identity that the majority of their caregivers may not know about. Therefore, when screening for screen time and social media use, clinicians should understand the bounds of confidentiality and when confidentiality needs to be respectfully breached. For example, if a child or teenager reports following diet trends on social media in an attempt to lose weight, a thorough history regarding disordered eating and compensatory mechanisms to lose weight should be taken. However, if a patient is not in significant medical or psychiatric danger, the clinician should only encourage the child or teen to disclose this information to the caregiver. However, if the patient is rapidly losing weight, utilizing laxatives or diuretics to lose weight, or is restricting their calorie count significantly, a caregiver should be involved and consideration for a higher level of care (eating disorder unit, adolescent medicine referral) should take place.

The Federal Child Abuse Prevention and Treatment Act (CAPTA) requires each state to have provisions or procedures for requiring certain individuals to report known or suspected instances of child abuse and neglect [78]. Currently, any sexting from a child to an adult is required by law to be reported to the respective children's services agency in the state in which the child resides [79]. However, sexually explicit images of children and teenagers shared, distributed, received, or kept by other children and teenagers is a relatively new phenomenon in the legal and professional realm of mandated reporting. Sexting laws are state dependent, meaning if a state does not have specific sexting laws, federal mandates and guidelines can apply and rely on child pornography laws [79]. Child pornography is considered a more severe crime than sexting, and therefore, clinicians should be aware of which laws apply in their state [80]. For example, in California, if a 15 year old sends a nude photo of themselves to a 17 year old voluntarily, and discloses this information to their mental health provider, California state law currently identifies such action as obscene sexual conduct of a minor and requires the clinician to report the action to their respective child service agency. In this scenario, the 15 year old is both the perpetrator and the victim, and if there was coercion or persuasion by the 17 year old to receive the text, they are also required to be reported by the clinician [79]. Highlighting what can be reported to child service agencies at the beginning of treatment relationships will help keep children and teenagers safe as well as prevent surprise breaches in confidentiality.

Regarding self-harm, mental health providers should be more well versed in when to report to parents about their children's safety. When children and teens disclose that they have been coming across images or text of self-harm on social media, clinicians should further explore what social media applications are providing this data and how it is affecting the teen. If the effects of contagion are leading to increasing thoughts of self-harm, clinicians should encourage the teen to disclose how they are feeling to their caregivers with clinician assistance. If the teen begins participating in self-harm or is distributing images of their self-harm online through social media platforms, clinicians should be informing the respective caregivers as well as developing a safety plan. At this point, safety needs to be prioritized over the therapeutic alliance.

Conclusion

Children and teenagers are living in the digital world. There is little uncertainty that screen time, social media use, and online interactions have increased over the decade, even more so during the COVID-19 pandemic. The smartphone has become the medium in which children and teenagers access each other. Furthermore, social media, through applications like Tiktok, Snapchat, and Instagram, have served as a bridge for teens to express themselves, connect with peers, and enjoy entertainment as well as educational content. However, with the expansion of technological innovation via virtual playgrounds, teens and children are also experiencing detrimental effects to their mental and physical health. Sleep deprivation as well as exacerbation of pre-existing mental illness such as depression and anxiety correlate with increased screen time use and social media exposure. Additionally, cyberbullying, sexual exploitation, and self-harm are also becoming more apparent dangers that children and teenagers face when they set their foot in a digital landscape. Our job as mental health providers is to screen and assess our patient's experience of the digital world and to do so, we need to continually educate ourselves of what our patients see when they open their phones.

Multiple Choice Questions

1. Per Common Sense Media, what percentage of U.S. children 11 and younger have access to a smartphone?
   A. 32%
   B. 46%
   C. 53%
   D. 72%

   Correct Answer: C. Pew Research conducted a study in 2018, examining smart phone use. Approximately 53% of children 11 and younger had access to a smartphone, which was much higher than the previous decade.

2 Social Media and Screen Time in the Clinical Interview: What to Ask and What It...

2. Which social media application originally developed popularity through the sending and receiving of digital pictures that vanished from user's accounts after 24 h?
   A. Tiktok
   B. Snapchat
   C. Instagram
   D. Twitter

   Correct Answer: B. Founded in 2011,Snapchat is a social media application that prides itself on a simple concept: any picture or video that a user sends is only available to the recipient for a short time before it becomes inaccessible. This feature has been now copied by other social media sites such as Instagram.

3. You are a clinician in California interviewing a 17-year-old patient who endorses sending and receiving nude photos from another 17-year-old teenager. They note that the act was consensual. What are your responsibilities as a clinician regarding mandated reporting?
   A. Report to the respective state child state service agencies.
   B. Do not report to respective state child state service agencies and parents as the patient notes that acts were consensual.
   C. Speak with parents about texting as intervention only as behavior can be mediated in an outpatient setting.
   D. Consider discharging patient from practice as they are engaged in child pornography.

   Correct Answer: A. In the state of California, minors sending nude photos to each other are considered a form of obscene sexual conduct and requires the clinician to report the action to their respective child service agency. In this scenario, the 17 year old is both the perpetrator and the victim. It is of the utmost importance that clinicians recognize their state laws and how to help educate their patients on safe and legal practices.

References

1. Twenge JM, Martin GN, Spitzberg BH. Trends in U.S. adolescents' media use, 1976–2016: the rise of digital media, the decline of TV, and the (near) demise of print. Psychol Popular Media Culture. 2019;8(4):329–45. https://doi.org/10.1037/ppm0000203.
2. Rideout V, Pai S. The common sense census: media use by tweens and teens. Commonsensemedia.org; 2015. https://www.commonsensemedia.org/sites/default/files/uploads/research/census_researchreport.pdf. Accessed 28 Jan 2022.
3. Nagata JM, Cortez CA, Cattle CJ, Ganson KT, Iyer P, Bibbins-Domingo K, Baker FC. Screen time use among US adolescents during the COVID-19 pandemic. JAMA Pediatr. 2022;176(1):94. https://doi.org/10.1001/jamapediatrics.2021.4334.
4. Rideout V, Robb MB. 2019 census 8 to 18 full report updated—common sense media. Commonsensemedia.org; 2019. https://www.commonsensemedia.org/sites/default/files/uploads/research/2019-census-8-to-18-full-report-updated.pdf. Accessed 28 Jan 2022.
5. Shevenock S. YouTube, netflix and gaming: a look at what kids are doing with their increased screen time. Morning Consult; 2020. https://assets.morningconsult.com/wp-uploads/2020/08/26113344/200858_crosstabs_EDUCATION_Parents_v2_LM.pdf. Accessed 28 Jan 2022.

6. Anderson M, Jiang J. Teens, Social Media & Technology 2018. Pew Research Center: Internet, Science & Tech; 2021, May 27. https://www.pewresearch.org/internet/2018/05/31/teens-social-media-technology-2018/. Accessed 28 Jan 2022.
7. Auxier B, Anderson M, Perrin A, Turner E. Parenting children in the age of screens. Pew Research Center: Internet, Science & Tech; 2020, December 17. https://www.pewresearch.org/internet/2020/07/28/parenting-children-in-the-age-of-screens/. Accessed 28 Jan 2022.
8. Bayindir N, Kavanagh D. Social—Global Web Index. Global Web Index; 2018. https://www.gwi.com/hubfs/Downloads/Social-H2-2018-report.pdf. Accessed 28 Jan 2022.
9. Kemp S. Digital 2020: Global Digital Overview—DataReportal—global digital insights. DataReportal; 2021, February 11. https://datareportal.com/reports/digital-2020-global-digital-overview. Accessed 28 Jan 2022.
10. Murphy E, Regan NM, Kim Y, Lavery M, Champion T, Kumar HV. Fall 2020 taking stock with teens—Piper Sandler. Piper Sandler; 2020, October 6. https://www.pipersandler.com/private/pdf/TSWTs_Fall_2020_Full_Report.pdf. Accessed 28 Jan 2022.
11. Media use by children younger than 2 years. Pediatric clinical practice guidelines & policies, pp. 1451; 2017. https://doi.org/10.1542/9781610020862-part05-years
12. Yu M, Baxter J. Australian children's screen time and participation in extracurricular activities; 2016, September. https://growingupinaustralia.gov.au/research-findings/annual-statistical-report-2015/australian-childrens-screen-time-and-participation-extracurricular. Accessed 29 Jan 2022.
13. Jago R, Stamatakis E, Gama A, Carvalhal IM, Nogueira H, Rosado V, Padez C. Parent and child screen-viewing time and home media environment. Am J Prevent Med. 2012;43(2):150–8. https://doi.org/10.1016/j.amepre.2012.04.012.
14. Hale L, Kirschen GW, LeBourgeois MK, Gradisar M, Garrison MM, Montgomery-Downs H, Kirschen H, McHale SM, Chang AM, Buxton OM. Youth screen media habits and sleep: sleep-friendly screen behavior recommendations for clinicians, educators, and parents. Child Adolescent Psychiatric Clin North Am. 2018;27(2):229–45. https://doi.org/10.1016/j.chc.2017.11.014.
15. Franchina V, Vanden Abeele M, van Rooij A, Lo Coco G, De Marez L. Fear of missing out as a predictor of problematic social media use and phubbing behavior among Flemish adolescents. Int J Environ Res Public Health. 2018;15(10):2319. https://doi.org/10.3390/ijerph15102319.
16. Carter B, Rees P, Hale L, Bhattacharjee D, Paradkar MS. Association between portable screen-based media device access or use and sleep outcomes. JAMA Pediatr. 2016;170(12):1202. https://doi.org/10.1001/jamapediatrics.2016.2341.
17. Lenhart, A. (2009, August 19). Teens and mobile phones over the past five years: pew internet looks Back. Pew Research Center: Internet, Science & Tech. https://www.pewresearch.org/internet/2009/08/19/teens-and-mobile-phones-over-the-past-five-years-pew-internet-looks-back/. Accessed 29 Jan 2022.
18. Published by Statista Research Department, W. A. S., Hootsuite, Datareportal, Kepios. Most used social media 2021. Statista; 2021, October. https://www.statista.com/statistics/272014/global-social-networks-ranked-by-number-of-users/. Accessed 29 Jan 2022.
19. Published by Statista Research Department. U.S. tiktok users by age 2021. Statista; 2022, January. https://www.statista.com/statistics/1095186/tiktok-us-users-age/. Accessed 29 Jan 2022.
20. Published by Statista Research Department, 28, J. U.S. Snapchat usage by age 2020. Statista; 2020, September. https://www.statista.com/statistics/814300/snapchat-users-in-the-united-states-by-age/. Accessed 29 Jan 2022.
21. Published by Statista Research Department, 28, J. Instagram: Age distribution of global audiences 2021. Statista; 2021, October. https://www.statista.com/statistics/325587/instagram-global-age-group/. Accessed 29 Jan 2022.
22. Piper Sandler I. Taking stock with teens—fall 2021 infographic. Piper Sandler®; 2021, October. https://www.pipersandler.com/1col.aspx?id=6217. Accessed 29 Jan 2022.
23. Ucciferri F. Parents' ultimate guide to tiktok. Common sense media: ratings, reviews, and advice; 2021, March 6. https://www.commonsensemedia.org/blog/parents-ultimate-guide-to-tiktok. Accessed 29 Jan 2022.

2 Social Media and Screen Time in the Clinical Interview: What to Ask and What It... 27

24. Herrman J. How TikTok is rewriting the world. The New York Times; 2019, March 10. https://www.nytimes.com/2019/03/10/style/what-is-tik-tok.html. Accessed 29 Jan 2022.
25. Elgersma C. Parents' ultimate guide to Snapchat. Common sense media: ratings, reviews, and advice; 2021, March 9. https://www.commonsensemedia.org/blog/parents-ultimate-guide-to-snapchat. Accessed 29 Jan 2022.
26. Milyan A. Snapmap: The good, bad, and ugly for parents. Screen Time; 2019, March 27. https://screentimelabs.com/snapmap-parental-controls/. Accessed 29 Jan 2022.
27. Beveridge C. How to use Snapchat: a guide for beginners. Social media marketing & management dashboard; 2021, December 17. https://blog.hootsuite.com/how-to-use-snapchat-beginners-guide/. Accessed 29 Jan 2022.
28. Elgersma C. Parents' ultimate guide to Instagram. Common Sense Media: Ratings, reviews, and advice; 2021, March 10. https://www.commonsensemedia.org/blog/parents-ultimate-guide-to-instagram. Accessed 29 Jan 2022.
29. Forsey C. How to use Instagram: a beginner's guide. HubSpot Blog; 2022, January 18. https://blog.hubspot.com/marketing/how-to-use-instagram. Accessed 29 Jan 2022.
30. Instagram. Introducing Instagram reels. Instagram; 2020, August. https://about.instagram.com/blog/announcements/introducing-instagram-reels-announcement. Accessed 29 Jan 2022.
31. Ballard J. Teens use these social media platforms the most. YouGov; 2019, October 24. https://today.yougov.com/topics/lifestyle/articles-reports/2019/10/25/teens-social-media-use-online-survey-poll-youth. Accessed 29 Jan 2022.
32. Alzougool B. The impact of motives for Facebook use on Facebook addiction among ordinary users in Jordan. Int J Social Psychiatry. 2018;64(6):528–35. https://doi.org/10.1177/0020764018784616.
33. Shaulova E, Biagi L. Social media usage in Finland. Statista; 2021, July. https://www.statista.com/study/37855/social-media-usage-in-finland-statista-dossier/. Accessed 29 Jan 2022.
34. Lenhart A. Teens, technology and friendships. Pew Research Center: Internet, Science & Tech; 2015, August 6. https://www.pewresearch.org/internet/2015/08/06/teens-technology-and-friendships/. Accessed 29 Jan 2022.
35. Spies Shapiro LA, Margolin G. Growing up wired: Social networking sites and adolescent psychosocial development. Clin Child Family Psychol Rev. 2013;17(1):1–18. https://doi.org/10.1007/s10567-013-0135-1.
36. Top categories on TikTok by Hashtag Views 2020. Statista; 2020, July. https://www.statista.com/statistics/1130988/most-popular-categories-tiktok-worldwide-hashtag-views/. Accessed 29 Jan 2022.
37. Forrester Analytics consumer technographics® US Youth Survey, 2021. Forrester; 2021, November. https://www.forrester.com/Forrester+Analytics+Consumer+Technographics+US+Youth+Survey+2021/-/E-SUS6711. Accessed 29 Jan 2022.
38. Rideout V, Robb MB. 2018 social media, social life: Teens reveal their experiences. Common Sense Media; n.d.. https://www.commonsensemedia.org/sites/default/files/uploads/research/2018_cs_socialmediasociallife_fullreport-final-release_2_lowres.pdf. Accessed 29 Jan 2022.
39. Rideout V, Fox S, Peebles A, Robb MB. Coping with COVID-19: How young people use digital media to manage their mental health. San Francisco, CA: Common Sense and Hopelab; 2021.
40. Blomfield Neira CJ, Barber BL. Social networking site use: linked to adolescents' social self-concept, self-esteem, and depressed mood. Austr J Psychol. 2014;66(1):56–64. https://doi.org/10.1111/ajpy.12034.
41. Escobar-Viera CG, Whitfield DL, Wessel CB, Shensa A, Sidani JE, Brown AL, Chandler CJ, Hoffman BL, Marshal MP, Primack BA. For better or for worse? A systematic review of the evidence on social media use and depression among lesbian, gay, and bisexual minorities. JMIR Mental Health. 2018;5(3). https://doi.org/10.2196/10496.
42. Booker CL, Kelly YJ, Sacker A. Gender differences in the associations between age trends of social media interaction and well-being among 10-15 year olds in the UK. BMC Public Health. 2018;18(1) https://doi.org/10.1186/s12889-018-5220-4.

43. Scully M, Swords L, Nixon E. Social comparisons on social media: Online appearance-related activity and body dissatisfaction in adolescent girls. Irish J Psychol Med. 2020:1–12. https://doi.org/10.1017/ipm.2020.93.
44. Wang J-L, Wang H-Z, Gaskin J, Hawk S. The mediating roles of upward social comparison and self-esteem and the moderating role of social comparison orientation in the association between social networking site usage and subjective well-being. Front Psychol. 2017;8 https://doi.org/10.3389/fpsyg.2017.00771.
45. Jiang S, Ngien A. The effects of Instagram use, social comparison, and self-esteem on social anxiety: a survey study in Singapore. Social Media + Society. 2020;6(2) https://doi.org/10.1177/2056305120912488.
46. Jang K, Park N, Song H. Social comparison on Facebook: its antecedents and psychological outcomes. Comput Human Behav. 2016;62:147–54. https://doi.org/10.1016/j.chb.2016.03.082.
47. Hale L, Li X, Hartstein LE, LeBourgeois MK. Media use and sleep in teenagers: what do we know? Curr Sleep Med Reports. 2019;5(3):128–34. https://doi.org/10.1007/s40675-019-00146-x.
48. Woods HC, Scott H. #Sleepyteens: social media use in adolescence is associated with poor sleep quality, anxiety, depression and low self-esteem. J Adolescence. 2016;51:41–9. https://doi.org/10.1016/j.adolescence.2016.05.008.
49. Cousins JN, Sasmita K, Chee MW. Memory encoding is impaired after multiple nights of partial sleep restriction. J Sleep Res. 2017;27(1):138–45. https://doi.org/10.1111/jsr.12578.
50. Ferraro FR, Holfeld B, Frankl S, Frye N, Halvorson N. Texting/ipod dependence, executive function and sleep quality in college students. Comput Human Behav. 2015;49:44–9. https://doi.org/10.1016/j.chb.2015.02.043.
51. Cohen-Zion M, Shabi A, Levy S, Glasner L, Wiener A. Effects of partial sleep deprivation on information processing speed in adolescence. J Int Neuropsychol Society. 2016;22(4):388–98. s
52. Perrault AA, Bayer L, Peuvrier M, Afyouni A, Ghisletta P, Brockmann C, Spiridon M, Hulo Vesely S, Haller DM, Pichon S, Perrig S, Schwartz S, Sterpenich V. Reducing the use of screen electronic devices in the evening is associated with improved sleep and daytime vigilance in adolescents. Sleep. 2019;42(9) https://doi.org/10.1093/sleep/zsz125.
53. Sampasa-Kanyinga H, Lewis RF. Frequent use of social networking sites is associated with poor psychological functioning among children and adolescents. Cyberpsychol Behav Social Networking. 2015;18(7):380–5. https://doi.org/10.1089/cyber.2015.0055.
54. Keles B, McCrae N, Grealish A. A systematic review: The influence of social media on depression, anxiety and psychological distress in adolescents. Int J Adolescence Youth. 2019;25(1):79–93. https://doi.org/10.1080/02673843.2019.1590851.
55. Thorisdottir IE, Sigurvinsdottir R, Asgeirsdottir BB, Allegrante JP, Sigfusdottir ID. Active and passive social media use and symptoms of anxiety and depressed mood among Icelandic adolescents. Cyberpsychol Behav Social Networking. 2019;22(8):535–42. https://doi.org/10.1089/cyber.2019.0079.
56. Schwartz MD, Costello KL. Eating disorder in teens during the COVID-19 pandemic. J Adolescent Health. 2021;68(5):1022. https://doi.org/10.1016/j.jadohealth.2021.02.014.
57. Kleemans M, Daalmans S, Carbaat I, Anschütz D. Picture perfect: The direct effect of manipulated Instagram photos on body image in adolescent girls. Media Psychol. 2016;21(1):93–110. https://doi.org/10.1080/15213269.2016.1257392.
58. Faelens L, Hoorelbeke K, Cambier R, van Put J, Van de Putte E, De Raedt R, Koster EHW. The relationship between instagram use and indicators of mental health: a systematic review. Comput Human Behav Reports. 2021;4:100121. https://doi.org/10.1016/j.chbr.2021.100121.
59. Zhu C, Huang S, Evans R, Zhang W. Cyberbullying among adolescents and children: a comprehensive review of the global situation, risk factors, and preventive measures. Front Public Health. 2021;9 https://doi.org/10.3389/fpubh.2021.634909.
60. Willard NE. Cyberbullying and cyberthreats: responding to the challenge of online social aggression, threats, and distress. Champaign: Research Press; 2007.
61. Tian L, Yan Y, Huebner ES. Effects of cyberbullying and cybervictimization on early adolescents' mental health: differential mediating roles of perceived peer relationship stress.

2 Social Media and Screen Time in the Clinical Interview: What to Ask and What It...

Cyberpsychol Behav Social Networking. 2018;21(7):429–36. https://doi.org/10.1089/cyber.2017.0735.

62. Copp JE, Mumford EA, Taylor BG. Online sexual harassment and cyberbullying in a nationally representative sample of teens: Prevalence, predictors, and consequences. J Adolescence. 2021;93:202–11. https://doi.org/10.1016/j.adolescence.2021.10.003.

63. The annual bullying survey—ditch the label. Ditch The Label; 2017, July. https://www.ditchthelabel.org/wp-content/uploads/2017/07/The-Annual-Bullying-Survey-2017-1.pdf. Accessed 7 Feb 2022.

64. Scribner H. Teens are creating 'Hate pages' on Instagram to bully and 'trash' their peers. Deseret News; 2018, October 15. https://www.deseret.com/2018/10/15/20655935/teens-are-creating-hate-pages-on-instagram-to-bully-and-trash-their-peers. Accessed 7 Feb 2022.

65. Dean S. Snap suspends anonymous Q&A apps Yolo and LMK after lawsuit over teen's death. Los Angeles Times; 2021, May 11. https://www.latimes.com/business/technology/story/2021-05-11/snapchat-suspends-yolo-lmk. Accessed 7 Feb 2022.

66. Weimann G, Masri N. Research note: Spreading hate on tiktok. Studies in Conflict & Terrorism. 2020:1, 10.1080/1057610x.2020.1780027–14.

67. Self-generated child sexual abuse material: youth attitudes and experiences in 2020 findings from 2020 quantitative research among 9–17 year olds. Thorn; 2021, November. https://info.thorn.org/hubfs/Research/SGCSAM_Attidues&Experiences_YouthMonitoring_FullReport_2021_FINAL%20(1).pdf. Accessed 7 Feb 2022.

68. Richards V. Kids have been sexting more in lockdown. What can parents do? HuffPost UK; 2020, July 30. https://www.huffingtonpost.co.uk/entry/kids-sexting-more-in-lockdown-advice-for-parents_uk_5f1ab94dc5b6128e68242a0c. Accessed 7 Feb 2022.

69. Responding to online threats: minors' perspectives on disclosing, reporting, and blocking findings from 2020 quantitative research among 9–17 year olds. Thorn; 2021, May. https://info.thorn.org/hubfs/Research/Responding%20to%20Online%20Threats_2021-Full-Report.pdf. Accessed 7 Feb 2022.

70. Pugachevsky J. Here's how to sext on Snapchat like a total pro. Cosmopolitan; 2021, November 1. https://www.cosmopolitan.com/sex-love/a27611587/snapchat-sexting/. Accessed 7 Feb 2022.

71. Wille M. Instagram makes sexting effortless with new Vanish mode. Instagram makes sexting effortless with new vanish mode; 2020, December 10. https://www.inputmag.com/culture/instagram-makes-sexting-effortless-with-new-vanish-mode. Accessed 7 Feb 2022.

72. Anderson M. A majority of teens have experienced some form of cyberbullying. Pew Research Center: Internet, Science & Tech; 2020, August 14. https://www.pewresearch.org/internet/2018/09/27/a-majority-of-teens-have-experienced-some-form-of-cyberbullying/. Accessed 7 Feb 2022.

73. FBI. Stop sextortion. FBI; 2019, September 3. https://www.fbi.gov/news/stories/stop-sextortion-youth-face-risk-online-090319. Accessed 7 Feb 2022.

74. Giordano AL, Lundeen LA, Wester KL, Lee J, Vickers S, Schmit MK, Kim IK. Nonsuicidal self-injury on. Instagram: examining hashtag trends: Int J Adv Counseling; 2021. https://doi.org/10.1007/s10447-021-09451-z.

75. Giordano A, Lundeen LA, Scoffone CM, Kilpatrick EP, Gorritz FB. Clinical work with clients who self-injure: a descriptive study. Professional Counselor. 2020;10(2):181–93. https://doi.org/10.15241/ag.10.2.181.

76. Klonsky ED, Victor SE, Saffer BY. Nonsuicidal self-injury: What we know, and what we need to know. Can J Psychiatry. 2014;59(11):565–8. https://doi.org/10.1177/070674371405901101.

77. Carson NJ, Gansner M, Khang J. Assessment of digital media use in the adolescent psychiatric evaluation. Child Adolescent Psychiatric Clin North Am. 2018;27(2):133–43. https://doi.org/10.1016/j.chc.2017.11.003.

78. Clay AL, Okoniewski KC, Haskett ME. Child abuse prevention and treatment act (CAPTA). Encyclopedia Child Adolescent Dev. 2020:1–10. https://doi.org/10.1002/9781119171492.wecad222.

79. Theoharis M. Teen sexting; 2020, September 8. www.criminaldefenselawyer.com. https://www.criminaldefenselawyer.com/crime-penalties/juvenile/sexting.htm. Accessed 7 Feb 2022.
80. Strasburger VC, Zimmerman H, Temple JR, Madigan S. Teenagers, sexting, and the law. Pediatrics. 2019;143(5). https://doi.org/10.1542/peds.2018-3183.

Introduction to the Virtual World: Pros and Cons of Social Media

3

Jennifer Braddock, Sara Heide, and Alma Spaniardi

Introduction

Social media refers to the collection of online platforms that allow users to share virtual content with one another. Social media originated in the 1990s and since then, the number of platforms has rapidly grown and become mainstream. Among the dozens of social media sites, it appears that the most popular platforms are Youtube, Instagram, Snapchat, and Facebook [1]. The majority of adolescents use these four platforms. Each of these four sites offers different features, with the common goal of interpersonal connection.

Some sites, such as Snapchat, offer intimate connections with friends. Other sites, such as Youtube, broadcast to the greater public. The type of content differs between sites as well. Facebook, for example, allows for text posts. The other sites mostly limit their content to pictures and videos. Sites differ in how permanent an individual's post is as well. Posts on Facebook, for example, exist on a person's profile forever, or until it is deleted. Alternatively, on Snapchat, posts are automatically erased after 24 h. Although these sites all began with different core functions, many of them have adopted additional features from their competitors (i.e., Instagram allowing videos after the success of Vine, and Facebook allowing temporary "stories" after the success of Snapchat). These sites give adolescents enormous opportunities to connect with others in a variety of different ways.

J. Braddock (✉)
New York University, New York, NY, USA

S. Heide
New York Medical College School of Medicine, Valhalla, NY, USA

A. Spaniardi
Department of Child and Adolescent Psychiatry, New York Presbyterian-Weill Cornell Medical College, New York, NY, USA

© The Author(s), under exclusive license to Springer Nature Switzerland AG 2023
A. Spaniardi, J. M. Avari (eds.), *Teens, Screens, and Social Connection*,
https://doi.org/10.1007/978-3-031-24804-7_3

As these platforms have expanded their functions, adolescents have increased their time spent on these sites. The Pew Research Center reported in 2018 that 95% of adolescents report having access to a smart phone and up to 45% report that they are online "almost constantly" [1]. When we compare these statistics to studies from just three years prior, we see that the number of adolescents with access to a smart phone was below 75% and only 24% of adolescents reported that they were online almost constantly [2]. This ~20 point increase in both of these domains just 3 years apart illustrates how quickly social media dependence is growing among adolescents. Based on this information, we can predict that this social media presence will become even more widespread in years to come. We will likely see the rise of new social media platforms as well, such as TikTok, an increasingly popular site that displays short videos and personalized content.

Benefits of Social Media

Social media has numerous positive and negative applications for adolescents. Many of the benefits of social media involve extensions of fundamental developmental processes and conflicts teens are navigating in their offline lives, such as identity exploration, building social connections, and establishing independence [3]. Social media allows teens to form and maintain friendships, seek social support, express creativity, discover new perspectives and ideas, increase learning opportunities, and take an active role in their health and well-being. Social media provides an avenue for adolescents to connect with others, explore their interests, and become adept at navigating their complex social worlds.

Communication and Social Connection

Social media provides a new channel for teens to connect with others, which can increase their sense of belonging and broaden their social networks [4]. The enhanced opportunities for connecting with friends even when they are unable to spend time together in person may help buffer against loneliness and boredom [5]. Additionally, social media may foster improvements in friendship quality by allowing teens to practice self-disclosure and active listening [5]. Adolescents even report that their friends' social media posts offer additional information about their emotions, which helps them to better understand their friends and in turn feel more closely connected to them [6].

Additionally, social media allows adolescents to stay in touch with friends and family who live far away or who have moved, which can be a positive way to bridge physical distance and allow connection to continue and flourish [4]. The removal of face-to-face contact may also help adolescents who struggle with shyness or social anxiety overcome the barriers to communication that typically prevent them from connecting with peers, which can reduce feelings of social isolation [4]. Further, by making it possible for adolescents to connect with a wider social network than

3 Introduction to the Virtual World: Pros and Cons of Social Media

would be possible offline, social media can help adolescents learn from new perspectives and develop tolerance and compassion for diverse groups of people [5, 7].

Social media can also connect teens who are part of marginalized groups, who may not have safe or supportive communities in their offline environments. For example, LGBTQ+ adolescents are able to explore their identities, discuss their experiences, and connect with others through online support networks [8]. Being able to express themselves authentically and receive validation from others who can relate to them can be especially protective against the elevated risk of depression and suicidality LGBTQ+ youth face [8]. This may be especially true for adolescents who reported feeling uncomfortable or unsafe discussing their sexuality with their offline family and friends.

Seeking, Receiving, and Providing Social Support

Social media provides adolescents with extensive opportunities to request, receive, and provide social support. Due to its constant availability, social media allows adolescents to immediately reach out to friends for support when they are going through a challenging or distressing situation [9]. Communicating with friends during distressing or challenging situations can help adolescents to refocus their attention, talk about their feelings, and request advice [9]. Further, adolescents can reach out to many people at one time through social media, which can help provide diverse perspectives and improve mood [9].

Adolescents with depression may turn to social media for support in order to connect with other teens with depression and to avoid stigma against depression or mental health treatment when sharing their stories [9–11]. One feature of social media that may encourage self-disclosure of highly personal and sensitive information is the option of anonymity on many social media platforms [11]. Anonymity on social media may allow teens who would otherwise refrain from talking about their emotions and experiences to share their stories, connect with others who can offer emotional support and hope, and discover new coping strategies [9]. Additionally, some teens seek social support on social media due to barriers to engaging with offline mental health resources, such as high financial burden or lengthy waitlists to meet with therapists or psychiatrists [12]. In these circumstances, teens may use social media as an outlet for talking through their feelings, verbalizing their needs, and coming up with actionable steps they can take to cope with the things they are going through.

Exploring Identity, Creativity, and Interests

Adolescents can also explore their interests and engage in creative expression on social media. Teens can use social media to browse or create content related to topics they are interested in, which can promote confidence and authentic self-expression [9]. Additionally, through discussions with other people who share their interests, they can learn more about things that are important to them while also enhancing feelings of belonging [4, 13]. A combination of identity exploration and online communication has been associated with a more coherent sense of self in adolescence, effectively helping teens learn more about themselves and practice engaging with other people [6].

Social media is also embedded with numerous opportunities for creative expression, which can allow adolescents to have fun and share their talents with others. Social media may provide inspiration for creative projects and help adolescents learn new skills, both of which can enhance well-being and increase confidence [13]. By collaborating with friends or strangers to create visual content on social media, adolescents can experience feelings of competence and foster social connection [5]. By allowing adolescents opportunities to explore their identities, social media can provide momentary entertainment and contribute to lasting personal confidence.

Educational Applications

Social media can be a beneficial resource for adolescents in their educational pursuits. Teens can quickly and easily connect with their classmates to collaborate on group projects outside of school hours, discuss class topics, and share ideas and perspectives when they do not fully understand an assignment [7]. This can help adolescents improve their grades, decrease stress related to schoolwork, and enhance their engagement with the things they are learning about. Some classes have incorporated social media frameworks into assignments through forums like class discussion boards. Not only can discussion boards help adolescents practice their written language skills by presenting their thoughts and opinions clearly, but they can also enhance their ability to thoughtfully respond to their classmates' perspectives and questions [7]. Furthermore, social media sites, such as Youtube, offer a wide breadth of educational videos that adolescents can use to help them in their studies. This might be especially helpful for teens without access to tutors or test prep resources.

Access to Health Resources

Social media can also help adolescents find health information and resources, which may promote taking an active role in their health and well-being [7]. Social media can provide opportunities to engage with health experts, find information about relevant health topics, and discover new resources to improve health and well-being. Adolescents can also engage with peers on social media to seek advice and discover new coping skills [9]. Furthermore, many scientists and health professionals have incorporated social media as a form of outreach. There is a multitude of videos on Instagram, TikTok, and Youtube by academics that transform complex concepts into understandable and accessible content. However, adolescents should be cautious

3 Introduction to the Virtual World: Pros and Cons of Social Media

when seeking health information online, as social media posts may sometimes contain misleading or false information. It is important that teens learn to critically interpret health information and identify reputable sources of such information before following any advice they encounter on social media [14].

Risks of Social Media

Despite the benefits associated with social media, there also exist several risks adolescents may encounter through social media use, especially if they are not adequately protecting their privacy online. Common risks adolescents may face on social media include cyberbullying, triggering content, and pressure to be constantly available to friends.

Cyberbullying and Harassment

Cyberbullying is one risk of social media that has gained substantial attention due to its association with emotional stress and poor mental health outcomes for adolescents. Cyberbullying involves the use of digital technologies to contact someone or post about them in deliberately hurtful or threatening ways [14]. Cyberbullying is often an extension of offline bullying, with many of the same dynamics and tactics at play. Cyberbullying can negatively impact academic performance, self-esteem, and social connections [14]. Adolescents experiencing peer victimization at school are more likely to be targeted online and to experience feelings of social isolation in response to invalidating responses from peers on social media [14, 15]. Additionally, cyberbullying can potentially worsen negative cognitions and internalizing behaviors in vulnerable teens.

Cyberbullying may be especially insidious due to the possibility of anonymity on social media, the ability for bullies to contact the victim at any time of day regardless of where they are, and the ability for information to spread quickly to large networks. Social media makes it possible for bullies to harm adolescents even when they are home, increasing the frequency of attacks and preventing adolescents from being able to disengage from their bullies [16]. Victims of cyberbullying may feel like they are never able to escape their attackers, because they may not be able to establish physical safe spaces as they might with offline bullying [9]. Teens expressed that even if they did not have social media accounts of their own, they weren't protected from the harmful effects of malicious posts being spread about them by their classmates on social media, because peers would discuss these posts in person at school [9].

Cyberbullying that takes place through social media also makes it possible to spread hurtful, embarrassing information or photos about a person rapidly and to a large audience, potentially increasing the impact of the bullying as it begins to play out in front of more peers [16]. Additionally, the hurtful or embarrassing content may be in the digital space indefinitely, which may cause an adolescent to feel as though they are being repeatedly victimized, because their peers can view harmful posts continuously.

Online disinhibition refers to the phenomenon where people may be more outspoken and less restrained online. This paired with anonymity may interact to expose victims of cyberbullying to more extreme, aggressive, and hurtful remarks and behaviors than they might experience in offline, traditional bullying [16, 17]. Anonymity allows a greater opportunity for people who are dealing with their own negative emotions to displace or project their negative feeling on others without fear of facing the same repercussions they would face if their identity was known [16].

Adolescents may encounter hate groups, discrimination, and hurtful comments on social media [8, 17]. Even complete strangers can contribute to toxic online environments through the process of online shaming, where people can upload photos or videos they took of people in public to social media to express contempt for their appearance or behavior [18]. Even if the person's behaviors were taken out of context, such posts can go "viral" and not only make it possible for a wider audience to collectively ridicule them, but also for the person to see the post themselves. Seeing that a post making fun of them was shared online without their awareness can be distressing enough, but the impact is amplified through hurtful comments added by other people and being confronted with complete strangers laughing at their expense.

Adolescents have also described how their private conversations can be made public through screenshots taken by peers and then shared to a larger audience than originally intended, which is associated with emotional distress and deteriorating relationships [16]. The ability for others to actively exclude teens on social media has also been associated with increased depressive symptoms, through such behaviors as blocking and deliberately cropping an individual out of a group photo, which can increase feelings of isolation [16].

Encountering Triggering Content

Social media may provide access to useful information for teens looking for resources to cope with challenging emotions and risky behaviors. However, adolescents have reported that one downside to seeking support through social media is that they may unexpectedly be exposed to triggering content, which can negatively impact their mood and even prompt relapses in behaviors like self-harm and drug use [19]. Triggering content can be emotionally distressing, unexpected, and at times impact an adolescent's ability to disengage from harmful behaviors. When triggering posts and photos are routinely encountered among other social media posts, it can also effectively normalize harmful and dangerous behaviors, and in some cases, even actively encourage it [11].

Due to correlates with depression and suicidality, self-harm is one topic of concern when addressing risky behaviors that adolescents might post online. Although it has been posited that exposure to such content can prompt a contagion effect, where viewers will begin to engage in the behavior themselves, research presents a more nuanced picture. In one study, posting, but not viewing, self-harm content was positively correlated with lifetime suicidality among adolescents who had recently engaged in self-harm [20]. For some adolescents, encountering graphic images of self-harm on social media can be especially upsetting when they are using social media to try to distract themselves from their own negative feelings [19]. However, for many teens, even more distressing than photos of self-harm were the narratives of emotional pain that accompanied them, because these stories activated familiar feelings in themselves that became overwhelming [12]. Additionally, teens who turned to social media communities centered around self-harm for support expressed that, while they found it incredibly helpful to connect with others who understood what they were going through, they sometimes felt that they needed to continue self-harming if they wanted to continue to receive this social support [12]. This could prompt more frequent self-harming behaviors in teens, because it can be complicated to separate the social support they are receiving from the risky behaviors they are engaging in [12]. Adolescents may post risky or triggering content on social media even when they are not truly comfortable with it, because it may ensure that they will receive attention and social support [19], with the consequence of normalizing behaviors that have detrimental outcomes on teens' mental health, well-being, and life satisfaction [12].

Encouraging High Risk Behaviors

In addition to the promotion of self-harm related behavior, social media might have a role in encouraging other types of dangerous behavior as well. Many adolescents may follow profiles that share content related to alcohol or drug use [6]. By seeing these behaviors by their peers or even role models, teens will witness the positive reinforcement that these behaviors have (through likes and comments) but will rarely see the negative consequences associated with these behaviors. Furthermore, users may exaggerate how often they are engaging in those behaviors in order to appear more mature or socially connected. As a result, risky behaviors may become more normalized amongst teens and thus may encourage their involvement.

Negative Effects of Social Media Communication

Although social media can be a positive way for adolescents to stay in touch with friends, social media communication may have some drawbacks as well. The ability to immediately reach out to friends may be helpful when participating in exciting conversations or requesting support, but it can also contribute to patterns of excessive communication that can be stressful for adolescents to manage [5]. Adolescents may feel pressured to be constantly available to respond no matter where they are, what they are doing, or how they are feeling, which can increase feelings of fatigue, frustration, and stress [5, 21]. Some researchers have found that after using social media, adolescents felt a decrease in closeness to their friends, an effect that persisted even among teens who reported relatively low levels of loneliness [22]. Conversations with friends may not be as intimate online as offline, which may occur as a result of adolescents limiting self-disclosure online out of fears of screenshots being taken of their private messages or posts [5]. Further, adolescents may feel resentment toward their friends after engaging in online conversations with them at inopportune times, such as when they were trying to sleep, complete their homework, or spend time with friends or family offline. Additionally, teens may feel frustrated with the way their friends use social media, which can prompt arguments and tensions within a friendship. For example, people may make negative judgments toward others who they believe are oversharing or seeking attention through excessive or uncomfortably personal posts on social media [19]. Not only can oversharing or attention-seeking posts generate frustration for adolescents who do not approve of their friends using social media for such posts, but these behaviors can therefore lead to feelings of social isolation and rejection for adolescents engaging in them, even from their friends.

Sexting

Sexting is another risky use of social media, and it involves sending sexually explicit images or messages through digital technologies. Sexting can be associated with offline risky sexual behaviors, and it may lead to legal consequences, even if it was originally consensual [14]. Among adolescents who report having engaged in sexting, many felt pressured into doing so. Additionally, even if a teen feels comfortable sharing a sexually explicit message with one person or a small group of people, they cannot control what happens to the photo or message after they've sent it. This may lead to an adolescent's photo being shared without their awareness or consent among a large group of their peers at school, which can not only be emotionally distressing, but can lead to school suspension, social ostracization, and bullying [7]. Because there is no way to guarantee a photo or message involved in sexting can ever be truly deleted, people may continue viewing, sharing, and downloading it perhaps indefinitely, which can make adolescents feel distressed, violated, embarrassed, and powerless [7, 14].

Sometimes, sexting can even lead to legal consequences. This is a complex issue, and legislators are continuing to debate how to handle cases involving adolescent sexting. Legal implications vary by state, with sexting leading to felony child pornography charges in some cases and juvenile-law misdemeanors in others [7]. Things become especially complicated when adolescents are victims of cybergrooming, where sexual predators have established trusting relationships with them in order to coerce them into sexting [4]. Predators misrepresent themselves by lying about their age, identity, and intentions, and adolescents may truly not have known who they were communicating with when sexting.

Privacy Concerns and The Digital Footprint

Social media use makes up one component of an individual's "digital footprint," which consists of information about their online activities. Because they may not fully understand how their personal information can be collected and used online, adolescents may not adequately protect their privacy on social media. Adolescents who share too much personal information on social media are at risk for receiving negative feedback from peers, identity theft, and stalking [23]. Additionally, adolescents may not understand that the things they post online may be effectively permanent, leading them to make thoughtless social media posts that have serious future ramifications [14]. They may share posts in the heat of the moment without pausing to consider the consequences, and if they have their accounts set to share posts publicly, these posts may potentially reach wide audiences [7]. Social media posts that portray inappropriate, offensive, mean, or illegal activities, even if the adolescent intends for such posts to be taken as a joke, can lead to expulsion from school or extracurricular activities and even negatively affect future job opportunities or college admissions.

Social Media and Comparison

During adolescence, issues of identity development and interpersonal connection become especially important, increasing teens' focus on the way they are perceived by their peers [3]. While a desire for peer approval may foster positive, supportive social connections, it also encourages social comparisons, which can have a substantial impact on self-esteem.

Social Comparison Theory and Social Comparisons on Social Media

Social comparison theory proposes that people engage in comparisons to others in order to evaluate, improve, and enhance their own abilities and opinions [24]. Such comparisons can differentially impact self-esteem depending on how frequently and to whom the comparisons are made. Upward social comparisons, or comparisons made to people who are better in some dimension, generally link with a reduction in self-esteem, likely by emphasizing a person's own real or perceived shortcomings [6]. Conversely, engaging in downward social comparisons, or comparisons to individuals who are worse in some dimension, has been shown to increase self-esteem.

Social comparison may be especially likely on social media due to salient comparison features that do not exist offline, like friend count and likes [25]. These features may effectively allow teens to directly compare themselves with their peers as a way of determining their overall popularity relative to others. Because this information, as well as all social interactions that take place on social media posts published to a user's profile, is also viewable to social media contacts, it may be especially impactful to adolescents, who are very attuned to indicators of social acceptance [15]. Additionally, social media platforms allow for a constant flow of interpersonal information, which generates more opportunities for individuals to engage in social comparisons [26]. Further, studies have shown that, while people do not generally present themselves dishonestly on their social media profiles, they do tend to emphasize positive aspects of themselves and their lives [3]. This trend has led to an overall positive skew in the valence of social media content users are exposed to when browsing through social networking sites. Taken together, these unique elements of social media may mean that not only do adolescents have increased opportunities to compare themselves to others through social media, but the people to whom they are comparing themselves seem especially better off than they are. This prompts a greater number of more extreme upward social comparisons and contributes to decreased self-esteem and increases in depressive symptoms [3, 25].

Although viewing others' curated and artificially positive social media profiles may contribute to reduced self-esteem, the selective self-presentation opportunities afforded by social media can have the opposite effect when a person is curating their own profiles. Adolescents' self-esteem was enhanced when viewing and editing their own social media profiles [27], an effect that was attributed to the emphasis on the positive qualities they chose to emphasize in their profiles. The asynchronous nature of social media allows teens the time and space to decide exactly how they want to present themselves, an opportunity that is not always feasible in offline interactions [27].

Subsequently, when looking at their own social media profiles, improvements in self-esteem may be a result of viewing the positive attributes they have chosen to include on their profiles. Adolescents are able to engage in identity exploration while simultaneously exercising control over the way they present themselves to others. To ensure they are perceived positively by peers, adolescents may select their best attributes and achievements to share on social media and leave out less appealing elements of their lives in a process known as impression management [25].

The ability to use social media for impression management can be very appealing, especially to teens who may struggle with social anxiety, as it gives them the time and physical space to decide exactly what they want to share with their peers. This can be a positive process, where they are able to share only what they feel most comfortable sharing. However, this is complicated by the fact that impression management can be tied to social comparisons on social media as well as increases in rumination [28]. Adolescents report that metrics such as "likes" on social media can cause them to compare themselves to others to judge how popular they are relative to their peers [19]. Individuals may use "likes" as a way to gauge whether their social media contacts seem to have a more positive or negative impression of them, and it can become stressful or even overwhelming when they do not receive an acceptable number of likes. Adolescents have reported that they sometimes feel pressured to get "enough" likes or receive a positive response on their social media posts, which can take away from the positive impacts of using social media to present a version of themselves they feel

3 Introduction to the Virtual World: Pros and Cons of Social Media

comfortable sharing with the world [19]. Some teens even report deleting their posts, other people's comments, or even their entire accounts if they feel it may be detrimental to the way their peers perceived them. They're essentially focusing more on the response (or lack thereof) than on the intrinsic reward they gain through sharing positive components of their lives and personalities.

The perceived success of posts and profiles does not just have an effect on intrinsic values of self-worth, but has extrinsic motivations as well. As profiles become more popular, they are often monetized by special media sites or third party brands. This practice gives adolescents even more reason to focus on social impression of them rather than their own impression of themselves.

Attribution Theory

Attribution theory explores how people explain the causes of other people's behavior [29]. Importantly, it has been shown that when judging the reasons for other people's behaviors, people tend to make more dispositional attributions, meaning they are more likely to assume a person's actions are due to underlying, stable personality traits, rather than due to situational factors [30]. This tendency to attribute other people's actions to their personalities may help to explain why adolescents judge others on social media to be happier and more popular than they are: when people post positively skewed highlights about their lives on social media in the absence of any additional information, people who view this content may be inclined to assume that these positive situations truly represent what they are like and how they really live [31].

This effect may be especially amplified in the context of following strangers on social media. In the context of following strangers, adolescents may not have any additional information about them to balance out the very positive social media persona they are exposed to. Conversely, they would be able to contrast their friends' posts with the information they have about what their friends are like offline and what their friends are going through, therefore prompting less upward social comparisons, and as a result, contributing to less negative self-judgments [31]. Following more strangers was found to be associated with greater depressive symptoms, and it has been proposed that this was prompted by social comparison processes.

The fact that not all social media platforms are reciprocal, meaning that adolescents are able to follow people who do not follow them in return [31], further increases the chances that they can be exposed to a great degree of social contacts they would never otherwise have encountered. This kind of parasocial, one-way relationship additionally means that the increase in potential comparison targets does not come with a commensurate increase in genuine social contacts who may provide support [19]. Although people may feel positively about sharing a curated version of themselves through their social media profiles, they may not keep this in mind when viewing others' profiles. They know they put forward a generally positive version of themselves on social media, but they may not assume the same is true about their social media contacts, meaning they may make the false assumption that their social media contacts post positive content, because they are happier, more popular, and more interesting than they are.

Opportunities for Therapy

Social media use is widespread among adolescents, and it is often a fundamental extension of their offline selves and behaviors as well. Because so much of the research involving the potential impact of social media use on adolescent depression is in its early stages, where causal connections and underlying mechanisms remain to be fully elucidated, specific recommendations are likely to continue evolving. As new technologies and social media platforms are developed, it will be important to evaluate the way adolescents use them to inform clinical recommendations [32, 33].

Social media may be a valuable platform to reach vulnerable adolescents to encourage them to seek mental health treatment, and it may also be useful in reducing the stigma around mental health and mental health treatment [34, 35]. Providing education about social media and identifying risky behaviors adolescents engage in online can encourage more positive uses of social media, and it may even be possible to incorporate social media models directly into therapy.

Education

The foundation of positive social media use in adolescence may begin with education about social media, privacy protection, and coping skills to employ in the face of challenging online interactions. Ensuring that internet safety and digital literacy is taught at home or school can be an effective way to prepare adolescents for the potential risks they may encounter on social media, which can help them avoid negative mental health outcomes [7].

Discussing risks of social media can help adolescents to make informed decisions about the ways they use social media. Additionally, to help mitigate the risk of depression and suicidality of cyberbullying, parents and clinicians can discuss the risks of cyberbullying, promote adaptive uses of social media, and encourage adolescents to seek support from trusted adults if they or someone they know is being cyberbullied [7]. Because many adolescents report that they connect with strangers online, it can be helpful to educate them about the risks of online exploitation, so that adolescents can learn to engage in discretion when connecting with strangers online [7]. Some connections to strangers may be completely harmless and foster a sense of social belonging, while others may be unsafe. There are numerous features on many social media platforms that may help to protect users from privacy or content concerns. Helping adolescents to manage the privacy settings on their social media accounts can ensure they are not sharing with larger audiences than they intend. Informing adolescents about features like "muting" words or phrases on some sites like Twitter can help them to reduce the likelihood of encountering triggering posts when they are using social media for entertainment or socialization purposes as well.

Importantly, social media safety programs should go beyond providing information about online safety and provide skills that adolescents can use when they encounter challenging or risky situations online. Risky online situations do not generally develop out of a lack of knowledge about such risks, but rather a lack of skills to deal with them [17]. To this point, in one study about the relationship between adolescents' skepticism toward advertisements and the amount of personal information they disclosed on social media, it was found that adolescents who reported awareness of marketers collecting and using their data in the advertisements they presented on social media actually shared more personal information online, and stated the benefits of receiving personally relevant advertisements outweighed the risks [36].

One social media literacy program about body image, dieting, and well-being, SoMe, taught adolescents to critique the content they encountered on social media and found it to reduce the negative impact of social media use on body image [37]. Additionally, educational programs about appearance ideals on social media were shown to be protective for adolescent girls against the negative effects of engaging in appearance comparisons on social media [38]. By showing teens side-by-side comparisons of unedited and edited photos, the potential impact of making comparisons on social media can be reduced, emphasizing the importance of informing adolescents that what they see on social media may not reflect real life to protect them from negative cognitions after using social media and feeling they do not measure up [38].

Identifying Risks and Encouraging Positive Use of Social Media

Social media is ubiquitous in adolescents' daily lives. Due to the potential associations it can have with adolescents' mental health, it is important for clinicians to ask questions about the ways teens use social media as well as the impact it has on their emotions. Because individual personality traits and life situations may interact with specific social media behaviors to determine whether social media has an overall positive or negative effect on adolescents' self-esteem, mood, and well-being, advice should center around specific social media behaviors that can be targeted to promote more positive social media use.

Some teens may be using social media in a primarily adaptive way, and even teens who are engaging in risky behaviors on social media can be guided to redirect their use in more positive ways [19]. By evaluating specific behaviors an adolescent is engaging in on social media, it may be possible to identify adolescents who may be at risk for developing depression [34]. For example, teens who report following a lot of strangers and engaging in more passive than active uses of social media may be at particular risk due to the potential to engage in frequent upward social comparisons. It can be helpful to inform adolescents that people generally present an unrealistically positive view of their lives on social media, so that they do not experience negative emotions related to comparisons to peers online [39]. Additionally, if teens follow a lot of strangers rather than friends on social media, it may be instructive to encourage them to interact more frequently with friends online [31].

In the context of a therapeutic relationship, encouraging adolescents to consider and discuss the way their social media use impacts their emotions can help to identify and practice new ways to think and behave in response to such emotions [40]. Additionally, because social media is often an extension of an adolescent's offline life, it may be helpful to address general maladaptive behaviors they engage in so that they can develop coping skills they will be able to employ whether confronting a challenge online or in the real world [7]. For example, if an adolescent turns to social media to avoid negative emotional states or feels social media is the only resource they have to alleviate loneliness, it may be important to address their general patterns of avoidance [40]. This may look like helping the adolescent learn to identify, experience, and express their emotions, or helping them find fulfilling ways to experience social engagement offline [40].

Clinicians can teach adolescents how to adapt the thoughts and feelings they have in response to negative reactions they experience to things they encounter on social media [41]. For example, positive cognitive refocusing encourages people to engage in positive thoughts when they notice themselves having negative thoughts. If a teen begins to have negative thoughts about their bodies after browsing through other people's photos on social media, they may be asked to instead identify things they like about their bodies, which can redirect their thoughts and prevent them from becoming too deeply entrenched in their self-image. This has been shown to be easy to teach and effective at reducing body dissatisfaction [41].

Clinicians can also help to improve adolescents' online resilience, or their ability to effectively handle negative situations they encounter online. For example, to reduce the negative impact of FOMO (Fear Of Missing Out) on adolescents' mood and self-esteem, clinicians may want to provide education about social media and FOMO as well as help adolescents practice skills and develop thought processes to use when they find themselves experiencing FOMO online [42]. Through this exploration, clinicians can help adolescents manage their expectations of themselves and their friends, challenge the anxieties that underlie their feelings of FOMO, help them cope with uncertainty, and learn to redirect compulsive behaviors, such as feeling the need to immediately check notifications they receive. This can prepare adolescents to manage negative emotions and develop new responses to FOMO during social media use.

Additionally, adolescents should be encouraged to engage in adaptive uses of social media if they tend to use social media while feeling upset. Adolescents can be

3 Introduction to the Virtual World: Pros and Cons of Social Media

encouraged to connect specifically with people who have been supportive to them in the past and to use social media as a creative outlet rather than less directed uses when they feel upset or lonely [19]. Additionally, it may be advisable for adolescents to unfollow or mute accounts on social media that frequently evoke social comparisons that make them feel badly about themselves [9].

Conclusion

Social media use is practically ubiquitous in adolescents and with it comes many pros and cons as described in this chapter. It is important for clinicians to understand the unique challenges in order to guide young people in their development. However, focusing solely on the negative aspects of social media is easy. It is necessary to recognize that social media can also provide a world of advantages that were not available to earlier generations. Bolstering the use of these attributes is an equally important goal of therapy as protecting against the harms.

Multiple Choice Questions

1. What time period was social media thought to have originated?
    A. The early 1980s
    B. The mid to late 1990s
    C. The year 2000
    D. Between 2010 and 2015
    Correct Answer: B
2. The theory that proposes that people engage in comparisons with others in order to evaluate, improve, and enhance their own abilities and opinions is:
    A. Attribution Theory
    B. Social Media Literacy
    C. Social Comparison Theory
    D. Positive Social Refocusing
    Correct Answer: C
3. Which of the following is true regarding encountering triggering content through social media?
    A. Self-harm narratives can be more distressing than images for teens.
    B. Only adolescents who are comfortable sharing their story post self-harm images.
    C. The contagion effect is not seen through social media exposure to self-harm images.
    D. Using images and narratives of self-harm in therapy is a good way to prevent adolescents from acting on their own self-harm urges.
    Correct Answer: A

References

1. Anderson M. Teens, social media & technology 2018. Pew Research Center: Internet, Science & Tech; 2018. https://www.pewresearch.org/internet/2018/05/31/teens-social-media-technology-2018/

2. Lenhart A. Teens, social media & technology overview 2015. Pew Research Center: Internet, Science & Tech; 2015. https://www.pewresearch.org/internet/2015/04/09/teens-social-media-technology-2015/. Accessed 25 Jan 2022.

3. Nesi J, Prinstein M, Prinstein MJ. Using social media for social comparison and feedback-seeking: gender and popularity moderate associations with depressive symptoms. J Abnormal Child Psychol. 2015;43(8):1427–38. https://doi.org/10.1007/s10802-015-0020-0.

4. Cipolletta S, Malighetti C, Cenedese C, Spoto A. How can adolescents benefit from the use of social networks? The iGeneration on Instagram. Int J Environ Res Public Health. 2020;17(19). https://doi.org/10.3390/ijerph17196952.

5. Winstone L, Mars B, Haworth CMA, Kidger J. Social media use and social connectedness among adolescents in the United Kingdom: a qualitative exploration of displacement and stimulation. BMC Public Health. 2021;21(1):1736. https://doi.org/10.1186/s12889-021-11802-9.

6. Uhls YT, Ellison NB, Subrahmanyam K. Benefits and costs of social media in adolescence. Pediatrics. 2017;140(Supplement_2):S67–70. https://doi.org/10.1542/peds.2016-1758E.

7. O'Keeffe GS, Clarke-Pearson K, Council on Communications and M. The impact of social media on children, adolescents, and families. Pediatrics. 2011;127(4):800–4. https://doi.org/10.1542/peds.2011-0054.

8. Berger MN, Taba M, Marino JL, Lim MSC, Cooper SC, Lewis L, et al. Social media's role in support networks among LGBTQ adolescents: a qualitative study. Sexual Health. 2021;18(5):421–31.

9. Weinstein E, Kleiman EM, Franz PJ, Joyce VW, Nash CC, Buonopane RJ, et al. Positive and negative uses of social media among adolescents hospitalized for suicidal behavior. J Adolescence. 2021;87:63–73. https://doi-org.proxy.library.nyu.edu/10.1016/j.adolescence.2020.12.003.

10. Dodemaide P, Joubert L, Merolli M, Hill N. Exploring the therapeutic and nontherapeutic affordances of social media use by young adults with lived experience of self-harm or suicidal ideation: a scoping review. Cyberpsychol Behav Social Network. 2019;22(10):622–33. https://doi.org/10.1089/cyber.2018.0678.

11. Yeo TED. "Do you know how much I suffer?": how young people negotiate the tellability of their mental health disruption in anonymous distress narratives on social media. Health Commun. 2021;36(13):1606–15. https://doi.org/10.1080/10410236.2020.1775447.

12. Lavis A, Winter R. #Online harms or benefits? An ethnographic analysis of the positives and negatives of peer-support around self-harm on social media. J Child Psychol Psychiatry. 2020;61(8):842–54. https://doi.org/10.1111/jcpp.13245.

13. Li S, Kiuru N, Palonen T, Salmela-Aro K, Hakkarainen K. Peer selection and influence: Students' interest-driven socio-digital participation and friendship networks. Frontline Learning Res. 2020;8(4):1–17. https://doi.org/10.14786/flr.v8i4.457.

14. Reid Chassiakos Y, Radesky J, Christakis D, Moreno MA, Cross C, Council On C, et al. Children and adolescents and digital media. Pediatrics. 2016;138(5):e20162593. https://doi.org/10.1542/peds.2016-2593.

15. Lee HY, Jamieson JP, Reis HT, Beevers CG, Josephs RA, Mullarkey MC, et al. Getting fewer "Likes" than others on social media elicits emotional distress among victimized adolescents. Child Dev. 2020;91(6):2141–59. https://doi.org/10.1111/cdev.13422.

16. Paulin M, Boon SD. Revenge via social media and relationship contexts: prevalence and measurement. J Social Personal Relationships. 2021;38(12):3692–712. https://doi.org/10.1177/02654075211045316.

17. Harriman N, Shortland N, Su M, Cote T, Testa MA, Savoia E. Youth exposure to hate in the online space: an exploratory analysis. Int J Environ Res Public Health. 2020;17(22):8531. https://doi.org/10.3390/ijerph17228531.

3 Introduction to the Virtual World: Pros and Cons of Social Media

18. De Vries A. The use of social media for shaming strangers: young people's views. IEEE. 2015:2053–62.
19. Radovic A, Gmelin T, Stein BD, Miller E. Depressed adolescents' positive and negative use of social media. J Adolescence. 2017;55:5–15. https://doi-org.proxy.library.nyu.edu/10.1016/j.adolescence.2016.12.002.
20. Seong E, Noh G, Lee KH, Lee J-S, Kim S, Seo DG, et al. Relationship of social and behavioral characteristics to suicidality in community adolescents with self-harm: considering contagion and connection on social Media. Front Psychol. 2021;12:691438. https://doi.org/10.3389/fpsyg.2021.691438.
21. Vanman EJ, Baker R, Tobin SJ. The burden of online friends: the effects of giving up Facebook on stress and well-being. J Social Psychol. 2018;158(4):496–508. https://doi.org/10.108 0/00224545.2018.1453467.
22. Pouwels JL, Valkenburg PM, Beyens I, van Driel II, Keijsers L. Some socially poor but also some socially rich adolescents feel closer to their friends after using social media. Scientific Reports 2021;11(1):1-15. https://doi.org/10.1038/s41598-021-99034-0.
23. Ellison NB, Steinfield C, Lampe C. The benefits of Facebook "Friends:" social capital and college students' use of online social network sites. J Comput Med Commun. 2007;12(4):1143–68. https://doi.org/10.1111/j.1083-6101.2007.00367.x.
24. Festinger L. A theory of social comparison processes. Human Relations. 1954;7(2):117–40. https://doi.org/10.1177/001872675400700202.
25. Appel H, Gerlach AL, Crusius J. The interplay between Facebook use, social comparison, envy, and depression. Curr Opin Psychol. 2016;9:44–9. https://doi-org.proxy.library.nyu.edu/10.1016/j.copsyc.2015.10.006.
26. Alfasi Y. The grass is always greener on my Friends' profiles: the effect of Facebook social comparison on state self-esteem and depression. Personality Individual Differ. 2019;147:111–7. https://doi-org.proxy.library.nyu.edu/10.1016/j.paid.2019.04.032 .
27. Gonzales AL, Hancock JT. Mirror, mirror on my Facebook wall: effects of exposure to Facebook on self-esteem. Cyberpsychol Behav Social Networking. 2011;14(1-2):79–83. https://doi.org/10.1089/cyber.2009.0411.
28. Bible J, Lannin DG, Heath PJ, Yazedjian A. An empirical exploration of materialism, social media, and self-stigma. Stigma Health. 2021;6(4):384–9. https://doi.org/10.1037/sah0000348.
29. Heider F. The psychology of interpersonal relations. New York, NYrk: Wiley; 1958.
30. Ross L The intuitive psychologist and his shortcomings: Distortions in the attribution process. In: Advances in experimental social psychology. Academic Press; 1977. p. 173–220.
31. Lup K, Trub L, Rosenthal L. Instagram #Instasad?: exploring associations among instagram use, depressive symptoms, negative social comparison, and strangers followed. Cyberpsychol Behav Social Networking. 2015;18(5):247–52. https://doi.org/10.1089/cyber.2014.0560.
32. Kreski N, Platt J, Rutherford C, Olfson M, Odgers C, Schulenberg J, et al. Social media use and depressive symptoms among united states adolescents. J Adolescent Health. 2021;68(3):572–9. https://doi.org/10.1016/j.jadohealth.2020.07.006.
33. Midgley C, Thai S, Lockwood P, Kovacheff C, Page-Gould E. When every day is a high school reunion: social media comparisons and self-esteem. J Personality Social Psychol. 2021;121(2):285–307. https://doi.org/10.1037/pspi0000336.
34. Ly L, Sidani JE, Shensa A, Radovic A, Miller E, Colditz JB, et al. Association between social media use and depression among U.S. young adults. Depression Anxiety. 2016;33(4):323–31. https://doi.org/10.1002/da.22466.
35. Memon A, Sharma S, Mohite S, Jain S. The role of online social networking on deliberate self-harm and suicidality in adolescents: a systematized review of literature. Indian J Psychiatry. 2018;60:384.
36. Youn S, Shin W. Adolescents' responses to social media newsfeed advertising: the interplay of persuasion knowledge, benefit-risk assessment, and ad scepticism in explaining information disclosure. Int J Advert. 2020;39(2):213–31. https://doi.org/10.1080/0265048 7.2019.1585650.

37. Gordon CS, Jarman HK, Rodgers RF, McLean SA, Slater A, Fuller-Tyszkiewicz M, et al. Outcomes of a cluster randomized controlled trial of the SoMe social media literacy program for improving body image-related outcomes in adolescent boys and girls. Nutrients. 2021;13(11). https://doi.org/10.3390/nu13113825.
38. Prieler M, Choi J, Lee HE. The relationships among self-worth contingency on others' approval, appearance comparisons on facebook, and adolescent girls' body esteem: a cross-cultural study. Int J Environ Res Public Health. 2021;18(3). https://doi.org/10.3390/ijerph18030901.
39. Li Y. Upward social comparison and depression in social network settings. Internet Res. 2019;29(1):46–59. https://doi.org/10.1108/IntR-09-2017-0358.
40. Bettmann JE, Anstadt G, Casselman B, Ganesh K. Young adult depression and anxiety linked to social media use: assessment and treatment. Clin Social Work J. 2021;49(3):368–79. https://doi.org/10.1007/s10615-020-00752-1.
41. McComb SE, Mills JS. Young women's body image following upwards comparison to Instagram models: the role of physical appearance perfectionism and cognitive emotion regulation. Body Image. 2021;38:49–62. https://doi-org.proxy.library.nyu.edu/10.1016/j.bodyim.2021.03.012.
42. Alutaybi A, Al-Thani D, McAlaney J, Ali R. Combating Fear of Missing Out (FoMO) on social media: the FoMO-R method. Int J Environ Res Public Health. 2020;17(17). https://doi.org/10.3390/ijerph17176128.

Social Media's Influence on Identity Formation and Self Expression

4

Maryann Tovar, Mineudis Rosillo, and Alma Spaniardi

Introduction

Adolescence is a time when young people strive for independence and separation from their family of origin. The ultimate goal of adolescence is the achievement of a unique identity. Conflicts between adolescents and parents are often directly related to this search for identity and include differences in core values, dress, and behavior. Friendships and peer relationships are of vital importance at this age, as acceptance and belonging to a social group are of central significance. The internet is a new arena in which adolescents can explore and test the limits of their identities. They are able to control and manipulate their digital persona in a way that may not reflect the reality of their "true" offline identity. This provides many opportunities for identity exploration, but also presents particular challenges and pitfalls. This chapter will discuss theories of identity development and apply these to the current digital landscape faced by adolescents today. We will also discuss the intersection of culture, race, sexuality, and social media.

M. Tovar
Department of Health Science, University of Carabobo,
Valencia, Carabobo, Bolivarian Republic of Venezuela

M. Rosillo (✉)
Department of Clinical Psychology, Bicentennial University of Aragua,
Maracay, Aragua, Bolivarian Republic of Venezuela

A. Spaniardi
Department of Child and Adolescent Psychiatry, New York Presbyterian-Weill Cornell
Medical College, New York, NY, USA

© The Author(s), under exclusive license to Springer Nature Switzerland AG 2023
A. Spaniardi, J. M. Avari (eds.), *Teens, Screens, and Social Connection*,
https://doi.org/10.1007/978-3-031-24804-7_4

Theories of Identity

Identity is defined as a subjective experience of who an individual feels they are and includes one's core beliefs, values, and goals [1]. A well-developed identity remains consistent over time. People who do not have a sense of who they are or their role in society can develop identity confusion. A main developmental task of adolescence is to explore and develop an individual identity, which will guide life choices during the transition to adulthood. Two major accepted theories of development pertaining to adolescence include Erik Erikson's Psychosocial Stages of Development and James Marcia's Identity Statuses.

Erikson's Stages of Psychosocial Development

Erikson's theory of psychosocial development includes eight stages from infancy to late adulthood (see Table 4.1) [2]. Each stage has a task, or conflict, which needs to be resolved in order to move on to the next stage. The tasks build upon each other throughout the lifespan and mastery of each one in sequence is required to continue moving forward. Successful completion of a task leads to competency and failure can lead to feelings of inadequacy. According to Erikson, the primary task of adolescence is to establish an identity through the task of

Table 4.1 Erikson's stages of psychosocial development

Stage	Basic conflict	Important Events	Outcome
Infancy (birth to 18 months)	Trust vs. Mistrust	Feeding	Infants develop a sense of basic trust if caregivers dependably meet their needs.
Early Childhood (2–3 years)	Autonomy vs. Shame and Doubt	Toilet training	Toddlers develop a sense of self-control and learn to do things for themselves.
Preschool (3–5 years)	Initiative vs. Guilt	Exploration Play	Preschoolers learn to initiate tasks and carry them out.
School Age (6–11 years)	Industry vs. Inferiority	School	Children apply themselves to tasks and learn to cope with social and academic demands.
Adolescence (12–18 years)	Identity vs. Role Confusion	Social Relationships Identity	Adolescents test roles and develop a sense of self-identity and personal identity.
Young Adulthood (19–40 years)	Intimacy vs. Isolation	Relationships	Young adults form intimate reciprocal relationships with other people.
Middle Adulthood (40–65 years)	Generativity vs. Stagnation	Work and parenthood	Adults have a sense of contribution and search for balance between productivity and feeling useful.
Maturity (65 to death)	Ego Integrity vs. Despair	Reflection on Life	Adults with success at this stage feel a sense of satisfaction and fulfillment when looking back at their life.

Identity versus Role Confusion. The core questions of adolescence include "Who am I?" and "Who do I want to be?" [2].

Erikson identified a period of psychological moratorium during adolescence, where committing to an identity is put on hold, while the young person explores options and experiments with different identities [3]. A stable and strong sense of identity marks achievement of the developmental task. Social isolation or becoming lost in the crowd can result from unsuccessful resolution of the task. In current times, identity formation is more commonly achieved later in young adulthood as opposed to during adolescence [4].

Marcia's Identity Statuses

Psychologist James Marcia recognized exploration and commitment as important factors in adolescent identity formation. He described four developmental identity statuses: diffusion/confusion, foreclosure, moratorium, and achievement (see Table 4.2) [5]. Identity diffusion refers to an individual who neither explores nor commits to an identity, while Identity Foreclosure is commitment to an identity without exploration of other options. Identity Diffusion is typically the status of children and young adolescents. A moratorium occurs during active exploration of options without commitment. Identity Achievement is when a commitment to an identity is made after the different options have been explored. Identity Achievement is often not achieved by the end of adolescence, but later into young adulthood. Unlike Erikson's stages, Marcia's statuses are not sequential and it is not necessary for an adolescent to progress through all the statuses to reach identity achievement. The theory also allows for multiple identity statuses simultaneously for different aspects of identity (religious, career, etc.) [6].

Table 4.2 Marcia's Identity Statuses

		Exploration	
		Low	High
Low	Commitment	**Identity Diffusion** There is no commitment and no motivation to question relevant issues.	**Identity Moratorium** Several options are explored, but no decision is made. Commitments are absent or vague.
High		**Identity Foreclosure** There is no exploration toward developing an identity, but instead identity is based on the choices or values of others.	**Identity Achievement** The development of a coherent and committed identity based on their own decisions.

The Digital World and Identity

Both Erikson's and Marcia's theories of development were conceived prior to the evolution of the internet; however, social media provides an additional multifaceted platform for adolescents to explore and experiment with their identities. The majority tweens and teens spend much of their day socializing via smart phones, computers, tablets, and other technology. According to a report by Common Sense Media, the amount of time spent on various individual screen activities increased by 42 minutes a day since 2015. Nearly 62% of youth spend more than four hours a day on screens and 29% use screens more than eight hours a day [7]. There are multiple platforms that adolescents can use online, including social media (Instagram, Facebook), online forums (Reddit), and group text messaging (Snapchat) The ability to curate an identity online is often easier than in the real world. In fact, many adolescents maintain multiple identities online across the same or different platforms.

In terms of defining an identity in the digital world, there are several ways of presenting yourself to others online. A *profile* refers to an online identity an internet user establishes on a website, social media, or online community. *Selfies* refer to photos that one takes of oneself, typically using a smartphone camera. As the name indicates, this is a self-portrait photograph, which can be used to represent an online identity when posted to a profile or can be used as an avatar. The use of photo filters further allows for personalization, or even falsification of one's identity. Photo filters range from the silly (adding rabbit ears or devil horns) to the more deceptive (adding a beard, glasses, or full face of makeup). The term *catfishing* on social media describes a person who impersonates someone else or creates a fake persona online to find friends or romantic interests. Usernames or also define an individual online. The names can be chosen to describe certain attributes, interests, or aspects of personality.

Adolescents can have multiple different social media accounts and maintain a different persona on each one depending on who their followers are. A teenager can share vastly different images and content across two or more accounts. For example, adolescents can present a more wholesome identity to family and friends while maintaining another account with different (sometimes more sexualized or inappropriate) content for close friends or strangers. Parents are unaware that they are following a "fake" account, while friends or strangers see a totally different side of their child. A common term for this is *finsta*, which stands for fake Instagram account, and it can also allow for a more anonymous way to interact online.

It has been found that having multiple online personas can be both positive and negative with regards to identity development. The freedom for self-exploration provided online can provide an adolescent the ability to express and accept different facets of themselves. Conversely, trouble in integrating these multiple self-representations can lead to a more diffuse and fragmented sense of self [8].

Anonymity Versus Exposure

The internet and social media can result in adolescents having to grow up in a more public way than ever before. The mistakes and missteps of youth can become a permanent part of their digital history. Relatives and friends have the ability to post pictures and information about the adolescent without their consent. At best, this visibility can cause youth to be cautious about what is revealed online. Adolescents can choose what is displayed [9], but also delete or *untag* material that others post. In this way, social networking can lead to increased self-awareness. Younger adolescents have been found to be more engaged in online impression management than older adolescents [10, 11]. This mirrors identity exploration, leading to eventual developmental achievements in identity formation.

There are many opportunities for adolescents to experiment with self-presentation online and to do this in an anonymous way. Anonymity on the internet is an opportunity for exploration and self-expression beyond everyday online and real life activities [12]. Anonymity can be freeing to adolescents in certain circumstances, but surprisingly can also result in an opposite, more restrictive online presentation. This is because an anonymous audience is unknown and less predictable, which can lead to self-consciousness and insecurity in the individual posting. It has been found that anonymity can be frightening and overwhelming for adolescents [13].

The ability to present oneself online without direct identifiers can lead to reduced self-awareness and decreased responsibility for one's actions, leading to online anti-social behaviors [14]. One example of this phenomenon is referred to as *trolling*. This term refers to a person who posts provocative, insulting, or offensive comments to purposely antagonize an individual or disrupt online communities. Another danger of online anonymity is being *catfished* or lured into a friendship or romantic relationship by someone who has fabricated an online persona. Often the goal of catfishing is for harassment or to scam or steal a victim's identity.

Adolescents display their real life persona in many social networking sites. Even when interacting on these platforms, which are not anonymous, they are aware that they are easily able to manipulate their true selves by hiding or changing certain aspects of their identity. This is often seen when teenagers change their name, location, or age. It is common for adolescents to label themselves as older than they really are in order to meet site age limits or interact with adults.

Online Versus Real World Identity in Minority Youth

On social media, it is possible to express and develop aspects of one's personality that is kept hidden in real world contexts. Since the internet has no geographical constraints, the opportunity for identity exploration and connecting with others is vastly expanded. This may be especially important for minority youth [15, 16] and can help to reinforce an individual's ethnic identity beyond their own environment [17]. When they create their profile on social media, they tend to emphasize the cultural aspects of themselves [18]. Similarly, sexual minority youth feel more comfortable expressing their sexuality online versus offline [19]. Despite this potential for freedom of expression, a study of adolescent girls identifying as sexual and ethnic minorities showed that they often hide their sexual identity on social media [20].

As a stronger more coherent identity is formed, aspects of self that have been explored online can be transferred to real daily life offline [21, 22]. It is an important step to be able to integrate views of online and offline identity into the real world. This change is evident in adolescents who start to present their real self on social media as opposed to using the platform for identity exploration [23].

Social Media, Self-Presentation, and Self Esteem

Friends and peer groups are very important during adolescence and expressing a certain image can solidify identity and belonging in a group. Self-presentation and learning social rules are developmentally important to preadolescents and adolescents. Social media adds another platform, and complexity, in which adolescents engage in *impression management*. This refers to the process of curating an online presence that gains peer approval [24–26].

Many young people are very savvy when it comes to social media self-presentation and maintain carefully crafted online personas. There are industries and professions created around online impressions, most notably *Instagram Influencers*. This refers to individuals who have built a reputation around a certain niche on Instagram. As the name suggests, they influence styles and trends. Young people often look to popular Instagram Influencers as guides as they explore their own identity. This can be problematic, as the lifestyle that is portrayed through social media sites rarely reflects reality, which breeds displeasure and negative self-evaluation when an adolescent uses their life as a comparison. Overall, the studies remain mixed in terms of social media sites and self-esteem, with some showing a positive effect and others a negative effect [27–29], as well as increased symptoms of depression and anxiety associated with social media [30].

The feedback that adolescents receive on their social media sites is closely associated with their experience online. This is likely due to the relationship between positive feedback on users' profiles and their self-esteem [31]. Social media feedback refers to *likes* given to a post by others on the network. This interpersonal feedback is often visible, either publicly or to the users' own network ("friends" or "followers"). It is common for an adolescent to check multiple times after posting on social media to see if others have "liked" the post. The stress of creating posts that gain enough "likes" as well as participating and "liking" the posts of friends can add up to a tremendous social demand and cause stress to adolescents [32].

Of course, not all feedback is positive. Instagram does not have a "dislike" option, but users can leave negative comments for all to see. Negative reactions on social networks are related to adverse outcomes, including depressive symptoms

[33]. Fortunately, positive feedback that is supportive and validating is more common than negative feedback on social sites [34]. The social validation received can result in an improved self-esteem [35], but paradoxically can create dependence on social approval, which is related to decreased self-esteem. Overall, the amount of feedback received can shape the identity development of adolescents [36].

The search for external validation, both in real life and online, can lead to a fragile self-esteem in teens and preteens [37]. The danger is when self-concept and self-esteem are tied to extrinsic traits, such as appearance or number of online followers. The goal of achieving extrinsic rewards and social validation seeking is negatively related to measures of well-being and self-esteem [38, 39]. Extrinsic rewards have also been found to decrease intrinsic motivation. The challenge is managing the fleeting social validation from "likes" and comments on a post, as well as the stress from constant comparison and search for perfection.

LGBTQ Identity Online

Identity development in adolescence naturally includes questions about sexual identity. Currently, there exist many recognized subcategories of sexual and gender identity, including pansexual and gender fluid. For Lesbian Gay Bisexual Transgender Queer Plus (LGBTQ+) youth, the internet and social media play an important part in the exploration of sexual identity, as well as provide information about sexual identity and health [40, 41]. The anonymity of the Internet allows adolescents to ask questions without feeling the stigma, shame, or discomfort that they might experience in real life [42]. There is also the opportunity to share experiences and obtain support from others in the community. Sexual minority youth can use social media to connect with others who are not geographically close. Video diaries or blogs can share personal stories of challenges or coming out which can provide comfort and support to those adolescents exploring their sexual identities. Many adolescents develop long distance romantic relationships and feel a strong bond despite never having met their partner in real life.

The internet allows adolescents to engage in relationships online that may not be available to them in real life. There are many opportunities online for people to connect, such as dating sites, instant messaging, chat rooms, and social networks. In regards to online relationships, studies have found that young people who are unable to disclose details about their personal lives in their real life often are involved in online relationships [43]. Online relationships can lead to positive connections with both heterosexual and homosexual peers, feelings of group belonging, and increased self-acceptance [44–46]. These relationships have a positive impact on LGBTQ+ youth's sexual and mental health, self-esteem, and quality of life [47].

Despite these benefits, research suggests that LGBTQ+ youth's internet use may also negatively influence decision making and offline behavior. A risk of close online relationships is decreased involvement in real life offline community and support systems, including friends and family [48]. There is concern that internet use fosters social isolation and depression. Research has also found that online dating is associated with unprotected sex and an increased number of partners [49, 50].

The Internet has played a critical role in facilitating identity exploration and coming out at a younger age. The development of a sexual identity can involve many questions, doubts, insecurities, and conflicts. For the young LGBTQ+ community, both the internet and social networks provide a platform to explore sexual identity and share information. The anonymity of these communities can be an advantage, since it allows adolescents and preadolescents to ask questions without a feeling of shame or discomfort that they might experience in real life. For young people belonging to the LGBTQ+ community, online relationships are often of great importance as they provide a space where they feel included and supported [47].

Cultural Viewpoint: Sex Education and Growing Up LGBTQ+ in Latin America

Growing up LGBTQ+ in Latin America can be challenging, as acceptance, education, and knowledge of gay rights are scarce. Despite the difficulties, this experience has been greatly improved and enriched by the presence of the internet.

Youth in Latin American countries are provided with few sources of information on sexuality or sex education. It is common that parents warn their daughters not to get pregnant after their menarche and encourage sons to look for as many girls as possible, but without bringing babies into the house. Latin America becomes the region with the second highest rate of unwanted pregnancies in the world, with around 18 percent of births corresponding to those under 20 years of age. One and a half million adolescent women between 15 and 19 years old have babies in the region each year according to UNFPA (The United Nations Population) [51]. Being able to access quality information via the internet provides education about safe sex practices to protect against pregnancy and sexually transmitted diseases.

In recent years, many organizations have raised their voices about the rights and freedom of sexual expression, and although progress has been made, the majority of the population of Latin America and the Caribbean "strongly disapproved" of same-sex marriage [52]. In Latin America, same-sex marriage is legal in 9 countries: Mexico, Chile, Cuba, Argentina, Brazil, Uruguay, Colombia, Ecuador, and Costa Rica. Argentina was the first country to enact a same-sex marriage law at the national level in Latin America, on July 21, 2010, while Chile was the country that most recently adapted its legal framework to allow these unions [53].

The LGBTQ+ community can encounter both positive and negative experiences online. There can be exposure to homophobic communities that present themselves under anonymity, but there are also networks that empower and create cultural and artistic support where the LGBTQ+ identity is safeguarded and enriched. Overall, the trend in attitudes toward homosexuality in both adolescents and adults in Latin America and the Caribbean has been more positive over the past ten years [52].

The internet provides a forum for young people to unite over shared ideals and goals to further LGBTQ+ rights.

Growing up in Latin America, being lesbian, gay, bisexual, transsexual, transgender, queer, can be a survival game, which unfortunately, many cannot win. Between 2014 and 2020, at least 3514 LGTBQ people were murdered in Latin America and the Caribbean. Of these, 1401 of them for reasons related to prejudice against their sexual orientation or gender identity. In 2019 alone, 327 cases were recorded during the 2020 pandemic, according to Sin Violence LGBTI [54]. Being able to connect with the online LGBTQ+ community provides support and a safe forum for those who do not feel comfortable expressing who they are in their real lives for fear of violence.

Latin America has a long way to go, but undoubtedly, the union of our efforts is what has allowed advancement in the education and promotion of rights and support for the most vulnerable communities. The ability for LGBTQ+ youth in Latin America to access information and join an international community is invaluable. This source bridges the gap in available information about sexuality and health that is greatly needed.

Clinical Application

It is important for mental health professionals and others working with children to understand the normal developmental stage of identity formation. This is a time of natural exploration and experimentation with different identities. The internet presents both advantages and challenges in identity formation and expression. Asking in an open and nonjudgmental way about a youth's online activities and personas can give much information about their inner life. This can provide for interesting material for psychodynamic therapy. It also allows for guidance and problem solving. It is important to discuss with young people the differences between real life and the reality presented by those online, who only show the high points or fabricate a perfect life. Although most adolescents understand this distinction, it is easy for them to fall into the social comparison trap, leading to feeling that their life or they themselves are lacking.

It is to be expected that an adolescent will not be necessarily forthcoming with the activities they are engaging in online. It is also common that they will withhold certain aspects to maintain their own privacy. Parents often have little to no understanding of what their child is doing online. Some are not interested, while others seem to avoid looking into it. That being said, there are families who are very involved in their children's online life. These families often have the agreement that children will share their online accounts and passwords with their parents. Online supervision is the best way to maintain safety. It is preferable to have teens be aware that their parents are monitoring and periodically keeping track of what they do online versus surreptitiously following their online activities. This is very family dependent, but therapists can guide families toward the appropriate level of supervision and facilitate open dialogues about expectations regarding internet use.

Youth who are questioning their sexual identity can be referred to websites that will provide them quality information and support as they explore. This is preferable to getting information from the internet at large, although as mentioned in the text, online communities and social support can be very important for adolescents. At the time of this printing, the CDC had compiled a list of LGBT youth resources including information for educators, professionals, family, and friends. This list can be accessed through the CDC website: https://www.cdc.gov/lgbthealth/youth-resources.htm [55].

Both Erikson and Marcia identify adolescence as a time of exploration. Young people have always naturally experimented and tried different identities during this stage of development. The internet and social media provide a vast new arena and allowing for this exploration to take place both online and offline. Issues of anonymity self-presentation, self-esteem, and consolidation of real-life and online self are important considerations. In terms of sexual identity and identification, the growth of the Internet has played a critical role in facilitating identity exploration and coming out at a younger age. Online relationships can lead to positive interactions with heterosexual and homosexual peers, greater social support, and feelings of belonging to a group. These elements can contribute to a positive self-esteem and self-identity. The anonymity of the internet allows young people to ask questions about identity and sexual health without feeling the stigma, shame, or discomfort that such questions can bring in "real life" interactions. As a result, online communities and support networks have grown in popularity. However, the negative aspects of these communities are episodes of identity crisis and negative influences in decision making.

Multiple Choice Questions
1. People who do not have a sense of who they are or their role in society can develop:
   A. Ego Integrity
   B. Identity Confusion
   C. Identity Foreclosure
   D. Identity Achievement
   Correct Answer: B
2. Which is true regarding the search for external validation online through seeking "likes" on social media posts?
   A. This type social validation builds a strong sense of identity.
   B. It can lead to a fragile self-esteem in teens and preteens.
   C. It is a cause of depression in all users of social media.
   D. There is no effect on any group of social media user.
   Correct Answer: B
3. Has the use of the internet in adolescents had a significant impact on the exploration of their identity?
   A. It has not had a significant impact as it inhibits young people from asking specific questions about identity and sexual health without the approval of a trusted authority figure.

4 Social Media's Influence on Identity Formation and Self Expression

B. It has not had a significant impact as young people only feel safe to express their concerns in an offline environment.
C. It has had a significant impact as it allows young people to ask specific questions about identity and sexual health without feeling the stigma such questions can carry in an offline environment.

Correct Answer: C

References

1. Kroger J, Marcia JE. The identity statuses: origins, meanings, and interpretations. In: Schwartz SJ, Luyckx K, Vignoles VL, editors. Handbook of identity theory and research. New York, NY: Springer; 2011. p. 31–53.
2. Erikson EH. Identity, youth, and crisis. New York, NY: W.W. Norton; 1968.
3. Erikson EH. Identity and the Life Cycle. New York, NY: WW Norton; 1994.
4. Cote JE. Emerging adulthood as an institutionalized moratorium: risks and benefits to identity formation. In: Arnett JJ, Tanner JL, editors. Emerging adults in America: coming of age in the 21st century. American Psychological Association; 2006. p. 85–116.
5. Marcia JE. Ego-identity status. In: Argyle M, editor. Social encounters. Penguin; 1973. p. 340.
6. Marcia JE. Development and validation of ego-identity status. J Personality Social Psychol. 1966;3(5):551–8.
7. Rideout V, Robb MB. The common sense census: media use by tweens and teens, 2019. San Francisco, CA: Common Sense Media; 2019.
8. Valkenburg PM, Peter J. Online communication among adolescents: an integrated model of its attraction, opportunities, and risks. J Adolescent Health. 2011;48(2):121–7.
9. Zhao S, Grasmuck S, Martin J. Identity construction on facebook: digital empowerment in achored relationships. Comput Human Behav. 2008;5:1816–36. https://doi.org/10.1016/j.chb.2008.02.012.
10. Strano MM, Queen JW. Covering your face on Facebook. J Media Psychol. 2013;24(4):166–80.
11. Jordán-Conde Z, Mennecke B, Townsend A. Late adolescent identity definition and intimate disclosure on Facebook. Comput Human Behav. 2014;33:356–66.
12. Keipi T, Oksanen A. Self-exploration, anonymity and risks in the online setting: analysis of narratives by 14–18-year olds. J Youth Stud. 2014;17(8):1097–113.
13. Suler J. The online disinhibition effect. Int J Appl Psychoanal Stud. 2005;2(2):184–8.
14. McKenna KY, Bargh JA. Plan 9 from cyberspace: the implications of the Internet for personality and social psychology. Personal Social Psychol Rev. 2000;4(1):57–75.
15. Boyd D. It's complicated: the social lives of networked teens. Yale University Press; 2014.
16. Spies Shapiro LA, Margolin G. Growing up wired: social networking sites and adolescent psychosocial development. Clin Child Fam Psychol Rev. 2014;17(1):1–18.
17. Markstrom CA. Identity formation of American Indian adolescents: local, national, and global considerations. J Res Adolesc. 2011;21(2):519–35.
18. Grasmuck S, Martin J, Zhao S. Ethno-racial identity displays on Facebook. J Computer-Mediated Commun. 2009;15(1):158–88.
19. Hillier L, Harrison L. Building realities less limited than their own: young people practising same-sex attraction on the internet. Sexualities. 2007;10(1):82–100.
20. Rubin JD, McClelland SI. 'Even though it's a small checkbox, it's a big deal': stresses and strains of managing sexual identity (s) on Facebook. Culture Health Sexuality. 2015;17(4):512–26.
21. Crowson M, Goulding A. Virtually homosexual: technoromanticism, demarginalisation and identity formation among homosexual males. Comput Human Behav. 2013;29(5):A31–9.
22. DeHaan S, Kuper LE, Magee JC, Bigelow L, Mustanski BS. The interplay between online and offline explorations of identity, relationships, and sex: a mixed-methods study with LGBT youth. J Sex Res. 2012;50:421–34. https://doi.org/10.1080/00224499.2012.661489.

23. Michikyan M, Dennis J, Subrahmanyam K. Can you guess who I am? Real, ideal, and false self-presentation on Facebook among emerging adults. Emerg Adulthood. 2015;3(1):55–64.
24. Chua THH, Chang L. Follow me and like my beautiful selfies: Singapore teenage girls' engagement in self-presentation and peer comparison on social media. Comput Human Behav. 2016;55:190–7.
25. DeAndrea DC, Walther JB. Attributions for inconsistencies between online and offline self-presentations. Commun Res. 2011;38(6):805–25.
26. Goffman E. The moral career of the mental patient. Psychiatry. 1959;22(2):123–42.
27. Gentile B, Twenge J, Freeman E, Campbell WK. The effect of social networking websites on positive self-views: an experimental investigation. Comput Human Behav. 2012;28:1929–33. https://doi.org/10.1016/j.chb.2012.05.012.
28. Gonzales AL, Hancock JT. Mirror, mirror on my Facebook wall: effects of exposure to Facebook on self-esteem. Cyberpsychol Behav Social Network. 2011;14(1-2):79–83.
29. Chen W, Lee KH. Sharing, liking, commenting, and distressed? The pathway between Facebook interaction and psychological distress. Cyberpsychol Behav Social Network. 2013;16(10);728 34.
30. Primack BA, Shensa A, Escobar-Viera CG, Barrett EL, Sidani JE, Colditz JB, James AE. Use of multiple social media platforms and symptoms of depression and anxiety: a nationally-representative study among US young adults. Comput Human Behav. 2017;69:1–9.
31. Valkenburg PM, Peter J, Schouten AP. Friend networking sites and their relationship to adolescents' well-being and social self-esteem. CyberPsychol Behav. 2006;9(5):584–90.
32. Weinstein EC, Selman RL. Digital stress: adolescents' personal accounts. New Media Society. 2016;18(3):391–409.
33. Davila J, Hershenberg R, Feinstein BA, Gorman K, Bhatia V, Starr LR. Frequency and quality of social networking among young adults: associations with depressive symptoms, rumination, and corumination. Psychol Popular Media Culture. 2012;1(2):72–86. *
34. Koutamanis M, Vossen HG, Valkenburg PM. Adolescents' comments in social media: why do adolescents receive negative feedback and who is most at risk? Comput Human Behav. 2015;53:486–94.
35. Stern S. Producing sites, exploring identities: youth online authorship. In: Buckingham D, editor. Youth, identity, and digital media. Cambridge: MIT Press; 2008. p. 95–117.
36. Clarke BH. Early adolescents' use of social networking sites to maintain friendship and explore identity: implications for policy. Policy Internet. 2009;1(1):55–89.
37. Manago AM, Vaughn L. Social media, friendship, and happiness in the millennial generation. Friendship Happiness. 2015:187–206.
38. Kasser T, Ryan RM. Further examining the American dream: differential correlates of intrinsic and extrinsic goals. Personal Social Psychol Bull. 1996;22(3):280–7. *
39. Georgiadis M, Biddle S, Chatzisarantis N. The mediating role of self-determination in the relationship between goal orientations and physical self-worth in Greek exercisers. Eur J Sport Sci. 2001;1(5):1–9.
40. Cohler BJ, Hammack PL. The psychological world of the gay teenager: social change, narrative, and "normality". J Youth Adolesc. 2007;36(1):47–59.
41. Savin-Williams RC. Identity development among sexual-minority youth. In Handbook of identity theory and research, Springer, New York, NY, pp. 671–689; 2011.
42. Suzuki LK, Calzo JP. The search for peer advice in cyberspace: an examination of online teen bulletin boards about health and sexuality. J Appl Dev Psychol. 2004;25(6):685–98.
43. Bargh JA, McKenna KY, Fitzsimons GM. Can you see the real me? Activation and expression of the "true self" on the Internet. J Social Issues. 2002;58(1):33–48.
44. Bargh JA, McKenna KY. The Internet and social life. Annu Rev Psychol. 2004;55(1):573–90.
45. Bargh JA. Beyond simple truths: the human-internet interaction. J Social Issues. 2002;58(1):1–8.
46. Boies SC, Cooper A, Osborne CS. Variations in Internet-related problems and psychosocial functioning in online sexual activities: implications for social and sexual development of young adults. CyberPsychol Behav. 2004;7(2):207–30.

4 Social Media's Influence on Identity Formation and Self Expression

47. Hillier L, Harrison L. Building realities less limited than their own: young people practicing same-sex attraction on the Internet. Sexualities. 2007;10:82–100. https://doi.org/10.1177/1363460707072956.
48. Boies SC, Knudson G, Young J. The Internet, sex, and youths: implications for sexual development. Sexual Addiction Compulsivity. 2004;11(4):343–63.
49. Liau A, Millett G, Marks G. Meta-analytic examination of online sex-seeking and sexual risk behavior among men who have sex with men. Sexually Transmit Dis. 2006:576–84.
50. Subrahmanyam K, Greenfield P. Online communication and adolescent relationships. Future Child. 2008;18(1):119–46. https://doi.org/10.1353/foc.0.0006.
51. Pan American Health Organization and the United Nations Population Fund, UNFPA 2020, Adolescent Pregnancy in Latin America and the Caribbean.
52. Latin American Public Opinion Project (LAPOP). Country questionnaires and sample designs <https://www.vanderbilt.edu/lapop/core-surveys.php>. Vanderbilt University.
53. Mena Roa M. Los países que le dijeron 'Sí' al matrimonio igualitario. Statista; Septiembre 27, 2022. https://es.statista.com/grafico/18091/paises-donde-es-legal-el-matrimonio-entre-personas-del-mismo-sexo/
54. Sin Violencia LGBTI (s.f.). Cifras De Violencia Contra Personas LGBTI En Latinoamérica. https://sinviolencia.lgbt/cifras-de-violencia-en-latinoamerica-contra-personas-lgbti/
55. Centers for Disease Control and Prevention (s.f). LGBT Youth Resources. https://www.cdc.gov/lgbthealth/youth-resources.htm

Fear of Missing Out: Depression and the Internet

5

Sara Heide, Jennifer Braddock, and Alma Spaniardi

Introduction

Major Depressive Disorder has become increasingly common among adolescents in recent years with 13% of U.S. teens reporting a depressive episode in 2017, up from 8% in 2007 [1]. Another statistic that is rapidly increasing among adolescents is their amount of social media use, with a 20% increase within three years [2]. These numbers have encouraged researchers to investigate a possible link between depression and social media use among adolescents.

Adolescent Depression

Depression is one of the most commonly diagnosed psychiatric disorders, affecting people of all ages. Despite the variations in emotional, physical, and cognitive maturity throughout the lifespan, the DSM criteria for diagnosing depression are mostly consistent among age groups. These criteria require patients to display five out of the following nine symptoms for a diagnosis of unipolar depression: depressed mood, decreased interest/pleasure in activities, significant weight loss or decreased appetite, insomnia or hypersomnia, psychomotor agitation or retardation, fatigue, feelings of worthlessness or guilt, diminished ability to concentrate, and recurrent thoughts of death [3].

S. Heide (✉)
New York Medical College School of Medicine, Valhalla, NY, USA
e-mail: sheide@student.nymc.edu

J. Braddock
New York University, New York, NY, USA

A. Spaniardi
Department of Child and Adolescent Psychiatry, New York Presbyterian-Weill Cornell Medical College, New York, NY, USA

© The Author(s), under exclusive license to Springer Nature Switzerland AG 2023
A. Spaniardi, J. M. Avari (eds.), *Teens, Screens, and Social Connection*,
https://doi.org/10.1007/978-3-031-24804-7_5

Although the diagnosis of depression must be objectively defined for practical purposes, depression likely exists on a spectrum rather than as a discrete entity [4]. Symptoms of depression may contribute to a diagnosis of unipolar depression, bipolar disorder, dysthymia, adjustment disorder, and many other psychiatric and medical diagnoses. Furthermore, this objective definition may lack sensitivity in certain individuals or demographic groups that display atypical or subclinical symptoms of depression. Additionally, the prevalence of depression may be underreported due to barriers to mental health resources and societal and cultural stigmas barring adolescents from proper diagnosis.

Despite these barriers in diagnosing depression, adolescent depression is estimated to be very prevalent in the population at 3.5% of children aged 12–17. This 3.5% is markedly increased from the 1.4% prevalence in 6–11-year-old and 0.5% prevalence in 3–5-year-old children [5] This trend, of increasing rates of depression throughout childhood, is a consistent finding among researchers. Some studies suggest up to a six-fold increase in rates of depression from early adolescence to the end of adolescence [4].

In addition to age, there is also a relationship between gender and depression. Studies have shown that female adolescents display higher rates of depression than their male counterparts. This relationship becomes significant in the ages of 13–15, as younger children display similar rates of depression between genders [6]. This female predominance persists into adulthood with a 2:1 female: male ratio [4].

Most people experience their first episode of depression during adolescence, and many of these individuals will continue to struggle with depression in their adult lives as well. The correlation between adolescent and adult depression is even more established than the relationship between childhood and adult depression [4]. There are many factors that may contribute to the high prevalence of depression in adolescents. For many, academic, social, and financial stress might become significant for the first time in adolescence. These environmental factors in the setting of a genetic predisposition contribute to the development of depression in many adolescents [4].

While there seems to be a relationship between adolescent and adult depression in the individual, it is important to note that clinical symptoms of depression may change throughout the lifespan. While adults typically experience a depressed mood, children and young adolescents may have an irritable mood instead [3, 7]. Irritability as a symptom of pediatric depression may result in the overdiagnosis of many behavioral disorders. For example, some researchers have found that the co-occurrence of ADHD and depression in youth is artificial when corrected for overlapping symptoms such as irritability [4].

Despite the very high prevalence of major depressive disorder, there is likely a large percentage of adolescents that experience symptoms of depression without meeting diagnostic criteria or being formally diagnosed. Considering this, it is important to examine adolescent self-reported depressive symptoms as well. It has been suggested that 20–50% of adolescents experience subclinical levels of depression [4]. These high rates of depression lead, in part, to very high rates of

5 Fear of Missing Out: Depression and the Internet 65

self-injury among adolescents. Rates of nonsuicidal self-injury range between 14% and 21% among young people, and rates of suicide have been increasing throughout the last decade [8], with suicide being the second leading cause of death among children aged 12–17 years in 2010 [5]. These numbers illustrate how much depression contributes to the morbidity and mortality of adolescents, irrespective of their formal diagnosis.

The etiology of adolescent depression is multifaceted with risk factors that include age, sex, and family history, as well as comorbid mental/medical illnesses [4–6]. Furthermore, the period of adolescence represents a vulnerable time in development, where variations in biology, genetics, personality, temperament, and cognition influence the risk of developing depression [4]. Given the high prevalence of adolescent depression, it is important to establish what modifiable factors are protective against depression and which increase risk.

One factor that has been heavily studied is the use of social media. Current adolescents are considered to be "Generation Z," as they were born between 1997 and 2012 [9]. This generation grew up during an unprecedented rise in internet and social media use. The internet allows incredible opportunities for education; however, it can also expose children to potentially harmful content. Similarly, the internet represents an opportunity to foster friendships while also increasing the risk that they will connect with potentially dangerous individuals. The complexity of the internet warrants a closer look into the role social media has on adolescents during this profoundly sensitive period of their development.

Internet Use Linked to Depression

While social media can act as an avenue to foster friendships, explore one's identity, and connect with like-minded individuals, there also exists a danger for adolescents to be exposed to potentially harmful content. Despite a growing body of research, there is not a clear consensus about whether social media is a contributing factor to poor mental health for adolescents. There are some studies that find no link between the two [10, 11]. However, other studies have suggested that there is a connection between social media and depression [12, 13]. These conflicting findings suggest that the link between social media and depression might be rather complex and require a more focused analysis to fully elucidate the relationship between the two. One such approach correlates symptoms of depression to different levels of social media usage: no usage, light usage (<1 h/day), moderate usage (3 h/day), or heavy usage (5+ h/day). When the data was analyzed in this way, the light users were highest in well-being and had more positive outcomes as compared to moderate or heavy users, but also as compared to nonusers [14]. This data suggests that the relationship between social media usage and depression might not be a linear one. This "U-shaped" relationship between social media and depression is a finding that has been corroborated by many other researchers as well [15].

Differences in Internet Use

The relationship between depression and social media is complex, likely nonlinear and influenced by a variety of different factors. Considering this, the link between social media and depression is likely very nuanced. A look into the different types of social media use may provide a lens through which to simplify the complex link between social media and depression.

Passive Versus Active Internet Use

One differentiation that has been described is the use of "passive" versus "active" social media [16]. This differentiates the passive viewing of posts from the active conversations held on social media. Some studies have suggested that active or directed interaction with friends is correlated to a decreased sense of loneliness [17]. Conversely, many studies have found that passive social media use is positively correlated to depressed mood, loneliness, and hopelessness and is negatively correlated to life satisfaction [18, 19]. This correlation likely relies on a greater likelihood for teens to engage in social comparison through passive social media use, while engaging in more protective activities such as social support with active social media use.

Feedback on Social Media

In addition to examining the different methods of social media use, another important factor that might influence the relationship between social media and depression is the type of feedback a user receives on social media. Social media involves more than just creating a profile and sharing personal information. It also allows contacts to directly respond to the content an individual shares. This interactive quality of social media, while providing an opportunity to build or strengthen social connections, may also impact the self-esteem of individuals through the general amount or valence of the feedback they receive [20]. In fact, it may not be time spent on social media, but rather the overall tone of the feedback adolescents receive online that determines social media's impact on adolescents' mood and self-esteem [20].

Receiving positive feedback on posts they share can help adolescents feel that they are accepted by their peers. Compliments from peers or comments on posts can make teens feel seen, supported, and appreciated. These feelings all arise from a sense that others are interested in them and that others have a generally positive impression of who they are as a person [21]. This sense of social connection and approval can be protective for adolescents' self-esteem and help mitigate the risk of developing depressive symptoms while using social media [20]. However, receiving negative feedback or not receiving feedback when it was expected both had negative effects on adolescents' mood and self-esteem [20]. When adolescents posted on social media with a specific hope for connecting with their peers and subsequently did not receive any reaction, they experienced increased feelings of loneliness and social isolation [21]. These feelings may prompt rumination in teens about potential reasons their social media contacts did not engage with them [22]. These effects may be amplified among vulnerable adolescents who already struggle with feelings of isolation, depression, or low self-esteem [23]. Beyond a lack of feedback, teens may also receive negative feedback on social media in the form of insults, invalidating remarks, or argumentative responses, all of which decrease self-esteem [20]. During and after receiving negative feedback on social media, adolescents may experience feelings of rejection, emotional distress, sadness, embarrassment, or shame, especially if they report placing greater importance on receiving feedback on social media [23, 24].

Friends Versus Strangers on the Internet

Another nuanced view through which to view the relationship between depression and social media usage is to look at what the relationships are between users. As discussed previously, different websites encourage different types of relationships. One of the major differences between Instagram and Facebook is that Instagram works through a "follow" system, whereas Facebook works through a "friend" system. A "friend" allows a mutual connection between persons where both parties view the other's content. In contrast, the "follow" system on Instagram allows one party to follow another without a reciprocal follow back. This system encourages users to follow profiles that they do not have a relationship with or know personally. One study revealed that higher Instagram use was correlated with greater depressive symptoms for those who followed more strangers, but lower depressive symptoms for users who followed less strangers [25]. This may be tied to the potential for more social comparisons made with strangers than with friends on social media. Essentially, while adolescents have information about their offline social connections that go beyond their positive social media profiles, they do not have such counterbalancing information about strangers they only know through social media [26]. By following more strangers, adolescents are potentially increasing their opportunities to compare themselves to individuals they do not have any offline information about. This potential relationship between following strangers and symptoms of depression is an important one to keep in mind when attempting to determine what types of social media usage might be harmful for adolescents.

The Effect of Personal Characteristics

In addition to the types of interactions adolescents are having online, the personal characteristics, such as gender, age, and personality of the users, might also contribute to an individual's risk of depressive symptoms.

Gender Differences

The greater incidence of depression in teen girls has been well documented. The Pew Research center has reported an almost three time increase in rates of depression among teen girls as compared to teen boys. While the incidence of adolescent depression is increasing for both boys and girls, the rate of depression in teen girls increased 66% between 2007 and 2017, while increasing 44% for boys in the same time frame [1]. Social media might act as a possible factor that influences this relationship between depression and the female gender in adolescents.

One study found that among girls who were at the lowest risk for depression, daily social media use was correlated to an increase in depressive symptoms. This same association was not found among teen boys [10]. One theory as to why this correlation exists might be the difference in exposure to negative influences online such as gender-based attacks and cyberbullying [27]. Although both boys and girls are at risk for negative interactions online, there is some evidence to suggest that girls experience more indirect forms of aggression, whereas boys experience more direct forms. This is hypothesized to result in a greater likelihood for girls to experience cyberbullying as compared to their male counterparts [26].Cyberbullying against girls can have devastating effects on their self-image and could result in depression in an already predisposed individual. Furthermore, there is also evidence that girls rely more on their social networks online, which may put them at particular risk for social isolation and feelings of loneliness when they experience conflict or harassment on the internet [28].

Age Differences

An additional factor to examine is age, and how it might affect social-media-related depressive symptoms. Younger adolescents might engage in social media in different ways and rely on different social media platforms than older adolescents. Parental monitoring of screen-use might also differ between younger and older adolescents, with older teens having less parental control. Social media sites often have minimum age requirements for users, but they commonly change over time. For example, Facebook was created as a site for college students, but has since lowered its minimum age to 13. Despite this, Facebook still remains more popular among an older demographic, in comparison to sites such as TikTok, which is increasingly popular among younger adolescents [29]. While Facebook encourages mutual "friendships," TikTok relies instead on the follower system. This might result in a greater likelihood that younger adolescents will interact with strangers, rather than friends on the internet.

Another difference between Facebook and TikTok is that while Facebook primarily shows the user posts from their friends, TikTok relies on a personalized algorithm, the "For You Page." As teens spend more time on TikTok, their "For You Page" becomes more personalized and begins to only show them content they enjoy or relate to. While this very personalized content might provide teens with a greater

5 Fear of Missing Out: Depression and the Internet

opportunity to connect with like-minded individuals, it also shields them from others who hold different beliefs or interests. For many teens, especially those from marginalized communities or with unique experiences or interests, this may result in them feeling a greater separation from friends and family off the internet who inevitably do not share all of the same attributes with them. In comparison to TikTok, Facebook shows the user posts from their friends, irrespective of the content they are sharing. As a result, older teens might be more likely to experience social connection to their loved ones by viewing posts about their lives, as opposed to only seeing content from strangers with shared interests.

The prevalence of cyberbullying also differs between age groups. It had previously been believed that cyberbullying peaks in middle school. More recent literature has suggested another peak in college-aged students as well [27], thus possibly leaving the youngest and oldest adolescents at the highest risk. Overall, age is a factor that can greatly influence the types of interactions a teen has online, as well as the type of content they view and the amount of cyberbullying they are exposed to.

Personality Differences

As adolescents spend more time on the internet, it becomes more difficult to control the amount of harmful content they are exposed to. Despite this, not every teen who is exposed to cyberbullying, social isolation, or upsetting content on the internet will develop symptoms of depression. The development of depression is influenced by many factors, many of which rely on the adolescent's ability to cope with negative experiences and avoid internalizing negative comments made about them on the internet. A factor that influences an adolescent's ability to do so is their personality type. In particular, some studies have found that certain personality traits such as neuroticism might be associated with an increased risk for depression [30]. Adolescents with neuroticism may have a decreased ability to cope poorly with stress and be more likely to experience emotional lability [30]. Interestingly, there has been some research to suggest that neuroticism is also linked to a greater immersion in social media [31]. In other words, adolescents with personality traits that include neuroticism may be more likely to be fully engrossed in their social media environment. This higher level of immersion in conjunction with a decreased ability to cope with negative emotions may put these teens at a particularly high risk of developing mood disturbances that are related to their social media use.

Associated Factors

While social media itself may have direct impacts on the mood of adolescents, it is possible that there are also many indirect factors that influence the relationship between social media and depression. These include quality of sleep, the act of multitasking, and level of physical activity.

Sleep

One possible indirect contributor to depression in social media users may be the relationship between depression and sleep. Many adolescents engage in social media in the evening, when they have more free time. This can result in staying up late, leading to a suboptimal amount of sleep for this age group [32]. Lack of sleep has a well-documented relationship to depression. It is probable that this relationship is bidirectional, but there is some evidence to suggest that many depressive episodes are caused or exacerbated by lack of sleep. This causal influence of sleep on depression has been established by studies that have noted an improvement in symptoms of depression with the treatment of insomnia [33]. Considering this, sleep disturbance might be one way that social media may influence the incidence of depression in young people.

Mutlitasking

Another possible associated factor is multitasking. Scrolling on social media is something that can be done without much active engagement. It is extremely common for adolescents to passively scroll through social media while they are involved in another activity such as watching television, having a conversation, or exercising. Interestingly, there is some evidence that increased multitasking is correlated to depression [12]. Additionally, some studies have suggested that an increase in media multitasking was associated with worse academic achievement, greater impulsivity, and poorer executive function [34]. Overall, media multitasking seems to have multiple negative effects on the cognitive function of adolescents, thus possibly contributing to the link between social media and depression.

Exercise

Exercise is another possible associated factor that might link social media to depression. There has been some evidence that social media's effect on exercise is nonlinear. It has been shown that among the physically active, social media use was positively correlated to physical activity. Conversely, for those who were not very active, sedentary behaviors were positively correlated to social media use. Users who were physically active at baseline likely followed exercise-promoting content, which further encouraged them to exercise. For those who were not active at baseline, social media use was likely associated with a decreased availability to spend on tasks such as exercising [15].

This relationship between exercise and social media is important, because there is a well-established link between exercise and depression. There are multiple different theories for why this relationship might exist, but it is likely multifaceted.

From a psychological perspective, exercise may be an intrinsic goal that an individual can work toward. Furthermore, exercise can act as a healthy distraction or an opportunity to connect with others. Additionally, there is a physiologic component as well, as exercise releases endorphins that might increase one's mood. For these reasons, exercise may be another indirect associated factor that links social media to depression. Interestingly, the relationship between social media and depression has been suggested to be "U shaped," which is the same relationship that has been found between exercise and social media. This provides more evidence that exercise might be a contributing factor to this relationship.

Related Cultural Phenomenons in Social Media

Social media is a relatively young entity, having been around since the 1990s. This new medium has brought with it unique related issues, which have made their way in the common vernacular. Of these, Facebook Depression and FOMO (fear of missing out) directly relate to mood.

Facebook Depression

One phenomenon that has attracted considerable media and research attention is referred to as "Facebook depression," [35] which refers to the development of depressive symptoms among adolescents who spend a lot of time on Facebook and other social networking sites. Research on the impact of Facebook use on adolescent mood has shown that in addition to believing their social media contacts are happier and more popular than they are [13], increased time spent on Facebook was associated with depressive symptoms.

Other researchers have found that more time spent on social media was not associated with a greater incidence of depressive symptoms in adolescents [11]. In fact, for adolescents with very low self-esteem, social media engagement may improve psychological well-being by promoting social connection and increasing social capital, or the resources one accesses through their social connections [36].

These equivocal results suggest that it is not social media use in general, but perhaps a combination of specific behaviors engaged while on social media and individual personality factors which determine whether social media use has a positive or negative impact on adolescent depressive symptoms. Among the factors commonly identified as potential mediators of the relationship between depression and social media use are: the amount and tone of feedback received on social media, following more friends or strangers, and the fear of missing out (FOMO); which all center around processes of social comparison. Social comparison is one key mechanism involved in the associations between social media use and depression. Such comparisons can impact self-esteem and self-worth.

FOMO: Fear of Missing Out

Social comparison is also tied to the phenomenon of the "fear of missing out," or FOMO. Social media posts can remind or show teens all the things they are "missing out on," which can lead to feelings of isolation, loneliness, and anxiety [25]. FOMO was found to be positively correlated with social comparison [37]. This may be exacerbated by the way in which social media is often viewed—during quiet or uneventful moments in their own lives [38]. Seeing posts or photos of peers having fun while they are engaged in things like completing their homework, trying to fall asleep, or feeling bored can really amplify the difference between what they are doing and what their friends are posting. This process may be similar to the way posts can prompt upward social comparisons. However, instead of just prompting negative appraisals of the self, FOMO goes a step further and may directly target feelings of loneliness and isolation, as well as lowered self-esteem. Seeing a post in which their friends are all out at an event without them may make them feel hurt, lonely, and as though they are unable to keep up with their peers [25].

FOMO can be very overwhelming to individuals, with some teens reporting that they feel obligated to remain connected to their phones just to avoid missing out on important updates from their friends [39, 40]. In the past, individuals would not have assumed that their friends were not communicating with them due to disliking them, but rather just because they weren't physically together. However, social media's constant availability can make FOMO especially likely [41], as teens may receive notifications directly to their phones at all hours of the day, making it challenging to disengage from social media. Furthermore, as social media becomes more prevalent among teens, there is an increasing pressure to always be within reach. In addition to using social media, adolescents use their phones and computers to communicate with their family or complete academic work. This can add another layer of difficulty when teens want to disconnect from the internet.

Social Media Models in Therapy

As more research is conducted on the relationship between social media use and outcomes such as depressive symptoms and self-esteem, it may become possible for specific interventions to be developed and utilized during the course of depression treatment. In fact, using online social media platforms as a component of mental health care may be a promising direction for treatment in adolescents, especially for those who enjoy using social media in their daily lives.

Social media sites may also serve as useful models for online mental health interventions. Some of the attractive features of social media, like immediate availability, the potential for anonymity, and peer support, may promote increased engagement in mental health interventions by youth who may otherwise be unwilling or unable to seek traditional mental health resources [42, 43]. Several studies have found that social media interventions may be helpful as adjuncts to traditional, offline mental health support as well as a standalone resource in preventing depression relapse in adolescents [42].

Research has shown improvement in symptoms of depression through a moderated online social therapy (MOST) model that integrates cognitive behavioral therapy approaches with social networking features [44, 45]. The MOST model includes features like self-guided therapy modules, moderation by clinical experts, and social networking components.

For example, the Rebound intervention was shown to improve depressive symptoms and prevent depression relapse in adolescents in partial or full remission [42]. Rebound included therapy modules focused on risk factors for depression relapse such as: rumination, self-criticism, and substance abuse; as well as behavioral coping skills to promote well-being including: self-compassion, relaxation techniques, mindfulness, and social connection. These modules were focused on providing psychoeducation to promote positive coping skills that could be applied in the adolescents' offline world. In addition to therapy modules, adolescents could turn to a moderated social forum on Rebound to propose topics for discussion and to request advice. Clinical moderators and other adolescents interacted on this forum to identify problems, brainstorm solutions, and discuss the pros and cons of various recommendations. However, in follow-up studies, two distinct groups of adolescents were identified in the Rebound study, one that preferred therapy content and one that preferred social networking content [43]. This emphasizes the importance of considering the adolescent's personal response to social media when determining whether a MOST model may be an effective component of therapy.

In another study, researchers found a slight decrease in adolescents' depressive symptoms after using a website called Supporting Our Valued Adolescents (SOVA) [46]. On SOVA, adolescents could view and comment on daily blog posts centered around themes of positivity, psychoeducation about depression and anxiety, information about social media platforms, and links to additional resources. This study showed preliminary evidence of using social media websites to promote peer support, decrease stigma surrounding mental health, and encourage adolescents to seek mental health treatment services. Importantly, adolescents expressed that they felt anonymity was central in their willingness to use the website and to disclose information about their feelings, an idea that may inform future moderated online social therapy sites.

Research has shown that it may be possible to develop interventions that are modeled after social networking sites with a specific focus on and promotion of mental health information. By incorporating a modality that feels accessible and fun for adolescents, such interventions can provide valuable psychoeducation and reduce the stigma surrounding depression and mental health treatment. This may also help to connect adolescents with supportive, informational communities that can buffer against the negative experiences and emotions they experience while depressed. However, studies have shown that user engagement can be an issue when implementing online mental health interventions [46], so it is important to check in with specific adolescents about whether they find such interventions personally helpful before recommending them.

Conclusion

Depression among adolescents is extremely prevalent and is a major contributor to the morbidity and mortality of adolescents. As social media use among adolescents rises, it is important to elucidate the role that social media might have in affecting the increasing prevalence of adolescent depression. While social media provides an opportunity for communication, learning, and self-exploration, there is also a great risk of cyberbullying, negative social comparison, and unsafe behavior. A growing body of research has suggested that the relationship between social media usage and depression is nonlinear and affected by multiple different factors. Some personal factors that influence this relationship are age, gender, and personality. Furthermore, the types of interactions online influence the correlation between depression and social media use as well. Active versus passive use, interacting with friends versus strangers, and receiving positive versus negative feedback are all elements that influence the overall net benefit or net risk that social media use gives to adolescents. Looking forward, possible interventions might include greater efforts to educate adolescents about online safety and encouraging their self-evaluation about the effects of social media on their mood. For clinicians, appropriately screening adolescents for high- risk internet behavior and providing them with targeted interventions accordingly will help to keep adolescents safe, while still supporting their social media use in a positive way.

Multiple Choice Questions

1. In regards to feedback on social media, which of the following was found to have negative effects on mood and self-esteem when adolescents post on social media?
   A. Receiving neutral feedback
   B. Receiving both positive and negative feedback equally
   C. Receiving negative feedback or not receiving feedback
   D. None of the above
   Correct Answer: C
2. What are examples of indirect factors that might influence the relationship between social media and depression?
   A. Sleep, frequency of multitasking, and amount of physical exercise
   B. Number of friends, quality of academic grades, and geographical location
   C. Family relationships, being vegetarian, and interest in computer programming
   D. All of the above
   Correct Answer: A
3. What is "Facebook Depression"?
   A. Low mood in the setting of not having a Facebook account
   B. Adolescents who like to present themselves as depressed on social media
   C. Having a low mood when one cannot access social media accounts due to technical difficulties
   D. The development of depression among adolescents who spend a lot of time on social networking sites
   Correct Answer: D

References

1. Geiger AW, Davis L. A growing number of American teenagers—particularly girls—are facing depression. Pew Research Center. 2019. https://www.pewresearch.org/fact-tank/2019/07/12/a--growing-number-of-american-teenagers-particularly-girls-are-facing-depression/. Accessed 25 Jan 2022.
2. Anderson M. Teens, social media & technology 2018. Pew Research Center: Internet, Science & Tech; 2018. https://www.pewresearch.org/internet/2018/05/31/teens-social-media-technology-2018/
3. American Psychiatric Association. Diagnostic and statistical manual of mental disorders (DSM-5 (R)). 5th ed. Arlington, TX: American Psychiatric Association Publishing; 2013.
4. Hankin BL. Adolescent depression: description, causes, and interventions. Epilepsy Behav. 2006;8(1):102–14. https://doi.org/10.1016/j.yebeh.2005.10.012.
5. Perou R, Bitsko RH, Blumberg SJ, Pastor P, Reem M, Ghandour D, Gfroerer JC, et al. Mental health surveillance among children—United States, 2005–2011. Cdc.gov; 2013. https://www.cdc.gov/mmwr/preview/mmwrhtml/su6202a1.htm. Accessed 25 Jan 2022.
6. Saluja G, Iachan R, Scheidt PC, Overpeck MD, Sun W, Giedd JN. Prevalence of and risk factors for depressive symptoms among young adolescents. Arch Pediatr Adolesc Med. 2004;158(8):760–5. https://doi.org/10.1001/archpedi.158.8.760.
7. Bernaras E, Jaureguizar J, Garaigordobil M. Child and adolescent depression: a review of theories, evaluation instruments, prevention programs, and treatments. Front Psychol. 2019;10:543. https://doi.org/10.3389/fpsyg.2019.00543.
8. Memon A, Sharma S, Mohite S, Jain S. The role of online social networking on deliberate self-harm and suicidality in adolescents: a systematized review of literature. Indian J Psychiatry. 2018;60:384.
9. Dimock M. Defining generations: where Millennials end and Generation Z begins. Pew Research Center; 2019. https://www.pewresearch.org/fact-tank/2019/01/17/where-millennials-end-and-generation-z-begins/. Accessed 25 Jan 2022.
10. Kreski N, Platt J, Rutherford C, Olfson M, Odgers C, Schulenberg J, et al. Social media use and depressive symptoms among United States adolescents. J Adolesc Health. 2021;68(3):572–9. https://doi.org/10.1016/j.jadohealth.2020.07.006.
11. Jelenchick LA, Eickhoff JC, Moreno MA. "Facebook depression?" social networking site use and depression in older adolescents. J Adolesc Health. 2013;52(1):128–30. https://doi.org/10.1016/j.jadohealth.2012.05.008.
12. Becker MW, Alzahabi R, Hopwood CJ. Media multitasking is associated with symptoms of depression and social anxiety. Cyberpsychol Behav Soc Netw. 2013;16(2):132–5. https://doi.org/10.1089/cyber.2012.0291.
13. Bollen J, Gonçalves B, van de Leemput I, Ruan G. The happiness paradox: your friends are happier than you. EPJ Data Sci. 2017;6:1–10.
14. Twenge JM, Campbell WK. Media use is linked to lower psychological well-being: evidence from three datasets. Psychiatr Q. 2019;90(2):311–31. https://doi.org/10.1007/s11126-019-09630-7.
15. Shimoga SV, Erlyana E, Rebello V. Associations of social media use with physical activity and sleep adequacy among adolescents: cross-sectional survey. J Med Internet Res. 2019;21(6):e14290. https://doi.org/10.2196/14290.
16. Primack BA, Escobar-Viera CG. Social media as it interfaces with psychosocial development and mental illness in transitional age youth. Child Adolesc Psychiatr Clin N Am. 2017;26(2):217–33. https://doi.org/10.1016/j.chc.2016.12.007.
17. Burke M, Marlow C, Lento T. Social network activity and social well-being. In: Proceedings of the 28th international conference on Human factors in computing systems—CHI '10. New York, New York, USA: ACM Press; 2010.
18. Krasnova H, Wenninger H, Buxmann P. Envy on Facebook: a hidden threat to users' life satisfaction? International Conference on Wirtschaftsinformatik; Feb 2013; Leipzig, Germany.

19. Aalbers G, McNally RJ, Heeren A, de Wit S, Fried EI. Social media and depression symptoms: a network perspective. J Exp Psychol Gen. 2019;148(8):1454–62. https://doi.org/10.1037/xge0000528.
20. Valkenburg PM, Peter J, Schouten AP. Friend networking sites and their relationship to adolescents' well-being and social self-esteem. CyberPsychol Behav. 2006;9(5):584–90. https://doi.org/10.1089/cpb.2006.9.584.
21. Cipolletta S, Malighetti C, Cenedese C, Spoto A. How can adolescents benefit from the use of social networks? The iGeneration on Instagram. Int J Environ Res Public Health. 2020;17(19) https://doi.org/10.3390/ijerph17196952.
22. Bible J, Lannin DG, Heath PJ, Yazedjian A. An empirical exploration of materialism, social media, and self-stigma. Stigma Health. 2021;6(4):384–9. https://doi.org/10.1037/sah0000348.
23. Lee HY, Jamieson JP, Reis HT, Beevers CG, Josephs RA, Mullarkey MC, et al. Getting fewer "Likes" than others on social media elicits emotional distress among victimized adolescents. Child Dev. 2020;91(6):2141–59. https://doi.org/10.1111/cdev.13422.
24. Nesi J, Prinstein M, Prinstein MJ. Using social media for social comparison and feedback-seeking: gender and popularity moderate associations with depressive symptoms. J Abnormal Child Psychol. 2015;43(8):1427–38. https://doi.org/10.1007/s10802-015-0020-0.
25. Lup K, Trub L, Rosenthal L. Instagram #Instasad?: exploring associations among instagram use, depressive symptoms, negative social comparison, and strangers followed. Cyberpsychol Behav Social Network. 2015;18(5):247–52. https://doi.org/10.1089/cyber.2014.0560.
26. Alfasi Y. The grass is always greener on my Friends' profiles: the effect of Facebook social comparison on state self-esteem and depression. Personality Individual Differences. 2019;147:111–7. https://doi.org/10.1016/j.paid.2019.04.032.
27. Kowalski RM, Giumetti GW, Schroeder AN, Lattanner MR. Bullying in the digital age: a critical review and meta-analysis of cyberbullying research among youth. Psychol Bull. 2014;140(4):1073–137. https://doi.org/10.1037/a0035618.
28. Ging D, O'Higgins NJ. Cyberbullying, conflict management or just messing? Teenage girls' understandings and experiences of gender, friendship and conflict on Facebook in an Irish second- level school. Fem Media Stud. 2016;16:805–21.
29. Auxier, Anderson. Social media use in 2021. Pew Research Center: Internet, Science & Tech; 2021. https://www.pewresearch.org/internet/wpcontent/uploads/sites/9/2021/04/PI_2021.04.07_Social-Media-Use_FINAL.pdf
30. Klein DN, Kotov R, Bufferd SJ. Personality and depression: explanatory models and review of the evidence. Annu Rev Clin Psychol. 2011;7(1):269–95. https://doi.org/10.1146/annurev-clinpsy-032210-104540.
31. Yu T-K, Lee N-H, Chao C-M. The moderating effects of young adults' personality traits on social media immersion. Front Psychol. 2020;11:554106. https://doi.org/10.3389/fpsyg.2020.554106.
32. Uhls YT, Ellison NB, Subrahmanyam K. Benefits and costs of social media in adolescence. Pediatrics. 2017;140(Supplement_2):S67–70. https://doi.org/10.1542/peds.2016-1758E.
33. Clarke G, Harvey AG. The complex role of sleep in adolescent depression. Child Adolesc Psychiatr Clin N Am. 2012;21(2):385–400. https://doi.org/10.1016/j.chc.2012.01.006.
34. Cain MS, Leonard JA, Gabrieli JDE, Finn AS. Media multitasking in adolescence. Psychon Bull Rev. 2016;23(6):1932–41. https://doi.org/10.3758/s13423-016-1036-3.
35. O'Keeffe GS, Clarke-Pearson K, Council on Communications and M. The impact of social media on children, adolescents, and families. Pediatrics. 2011;127(4):800–4. https://doi.org/10.1542/peds.2011-0054.
36. Ellison NB, Steinfield C, Lampe C. The benefits of facebook "friends:" social capital and college students' use of online social network sites. J Computer-Mediated Commun. 2007;12(4):1143–68. https://doi.org/10.1111/j.1083-6101.2007.00367.x.
37. Tandon A, Dhir A, Talwar S, Kaur P, Mäntymäki M. Dark consequences of social media-induced fear of missing out (FoMO): Social media stalking, comparisons, and fatigue. Technol Forecasting Social Change. 2021;171:120931. https://doi.org/10.1016/j.techfore.2021.120931.

38. Midgley C, Thai S, Lockwood P, Kovacheff C, Page-Gould E. When every day is a high school reunion: Social media comparisons and self-esteem. J Personal Social Psychol. 2021;121(2):285–307. https://doi.org/10.1037/pspi0000336.
39. Weinstein E, Kleiman EM, Franz PJ, Joyce VW, Nash CC, Buonopane RJ, et al. Positive and negative uses of social media among adolescents hospitalized for suicidal behavior. J Adolescence. 2021;87:63–73. https://doi.org/10.1016/j.adolescence.2020.12.003.
40. Winstone L, Mars B, Haworth CMA, Kidger J. Social media use and social connectedness among adolescents in the United Kingdom: a qualitative exploration of displacement and stimulation. BMC Public Health. 2021;21(1):1736. https://doi.org/10.1186/s12889-021-11802-9.
41. Alutaybi A, Al-Thani D, McAlaney J, Ali R. Combating Fear of Missing Out (FoMO) on social media: the FoMO-R method. Int J Environ Res Public Health. 2020;17(17). https://doi.org/10.3390/ijerph17176128.
42. Rice S, Gleeson J, Davey C, Hetrick S, Parker A, Lederman R, et al. Moderated online social therapy for depression relapse prevention in young people: pilot study of a 'next generation' online intervention. Early Interven Psychiatry. 2018;12(4):613–25. https://doi.org/10.1111/eip.12354.
43. Santesteban-Echarri O, Rice S, Wadley G, Lederman R, D'Alfonso S, Russon P, et al. A next-generation social media-based relapse prevention intervention for youth depression: qualitative data on user experience outcomes for social networking, safety, and clinical benefit. Internet Interv. 2017;9:65–73. https://doi.org/10.1016/j.invent.2017.06.002.
44. Lederman R, Wadley G, Gleeson J, Bendall S, Álvarez-Jiménez M. Moderated online social therapy: Designing and evaluating technology for mental health. ACM Trans Comput-Hum Interact. 2014;21(1):Article 5. https://doi.org/10.1145/2513179.
45. Wadley G, Lederman R, Gleeson J, Alvarez-Jimenez M. Participatory design of an online therapy for youth mental health. Proceedings of the 25th Australian computer-human interaction conference: augmentation, application, innovation, collaboration. Adelaide, Australia: Association for Computing Machinery; 2013. p. 517–26.
46. Radovic A, Gmelin T, Hua J, Long C, Stein BD, Miller E. Supporting Our Valued Adolescents (SOVA), a social media website for adolescents with depression and/or anxiety: technological feasibility, usability, and acceptability study. JMIR Ment Health. 2018;5(1):e17. https://doi.org/10.2196/mental.9441.

Social Media and Cyberbullying

6

Jenna Margolis and Dinara Amanbekova

Introduction and Definitions

Bullying is an aggressive, willful act carried out repeatedly by a group or an individual against a victim who cannot easily defend themselves [1]. Traditionally, bullying can be direct—physical, verbal, or relational (e.g., social exclusion)—or indirect (e.g., rumor spreading). However, with the advent of electronic communication (e.g., social media and instant messaging), the internet, and mobile phones, cyberbullying has emerged as its newest form. Cyberbullying is defined as deliberate harmful behavior, carried out repeatedly, where there is a perceived or actual imbalance in power against a target who is vulnerable or cannot easily stand up to the perpetrator, inflicted through the use of computers, cell phones, and other electronic devices [2]. As will be discussed throughout the chapter, defining and understanding cyberbullying is complicated by the fact that cyberbullying can take many different forms and occur through so many different mediums. Researchers are working continuously to create definitions for cybervictimization that will help to better distinguish it from traditional bullying [3].

Cyberbullying can occur through a variety of venues including text messaging and messaging apps, instant messaging, direct messaging, online forums, chat rooms, message boards (e.g., Reddit), email, the online gaming community, and social media, such as Facebook, Instagram, Snapchat, Twitter, TikTok, YouTube, Yik Yak, WeChat and others [4]. Cyberbullying can include sending, posting, or sharing negative, harmful, false, or malicious content about someone else. Cyberbullying can be considered a crime if it involves making violent or death threats, stalking, sexting or sexual exploitation, child pornography, expressing hate crimes, and posting or taking a picture of someone in a place where they expect privacy [5].

J. Margolis (✉) · D. Amanbekova
Department of Child and Adolescent Psychiatry, NYU Child Study Center, NYU Grossman School of Medicine, New York, NY, USA

© The Author(s), under exclusive license to Springer Nature Switzerland AG 2023
A. Spaniardi, J. M. Avari (eds.), *Teens, Screens, and Social Connection*,
https://doi.org/10.1007/978-3-031-24804-7_6

Three forms of cyberbullying have been cited: (1) cyberbullying victimization, or receiving negative electronic communications; (2) cyberbullying perpetration, or initiating harmful electronic communications; and, (3) being a bystander who is witness to cyberbullying [6]. Studies have shown that being a cyberbullying victim is highly correlated with being a perpetrator. One theory behind this is related to the ability of cyberbullying victims to respond in real-time during online interactions. Once targeted, cyberbullying victims will often retaliate and then, in turn, become cyberbullying perpetrators. Similarly, bystanders may inadvertently pass along cyberbullying messages or respond in ways that are harmful to a victim, thereby also becoming perpetrators in their own right. In addition, studies have shown cyberbullying victims and perpetrators are also more likely to be involved in traditional victimization and perpetration [7]. Individuals can play multiple roles on social media, whether as victims, perpetrators, or bystanders. "Liking," "sharing," and "commenting" allows individuals to move from one role to another. Also, given the ability to respond live in online communications, cyberbullying victims often strike back and become perpetrators themselves.

While all cyberbullying takes place using digital technology, the ways acts of cyberbullying can be carried out are quite different, and youth report that the level of distress they experience fluctuates depending on the type of cyberbullying carried out [8]. For example, some perpetrators may befriend a target in order to gain personal information about them, just to later create incriminating public posts about the personal information shared (trickery). Others may try to find out the victim's password to a social media account and then login and create embarrassing or incriminating posts (fraping). Within the context of cyberbullying, there is the additional element of anonymity, which is also of particular concern. A common modality of cyberbullying is when a perpetrator creates a fake Instagram account (or a FINSTA) and then posts rumors or unflattering pictures of the target (impersonation). Anonymous posts about an individual can generate considerable fear on the part of the victim, as they are unsure who created these posts. Victims can find themselves suspecting everyone, which can cause significant harm to their relationships. Research has shown denigration, outing, trickery, exclusion, and masquerading are the most distressing for children, while sending or distributing sexual images was the most upsetting for college students [8]. The various subtypes of cyberbullying are described in Fig. 6.1.

Cyber-aggression, which more broadly describes negative internet behaviors, should be distinguished from cyberbullying. In cyber-aggression, the interaction occurs either occasionally or as a one-off occurrence, and is communicated between people or groups of people where there may not be a power imbalance. It also may not include an intention to inflict harm or distress. An example of this may be an individual responding rudely to a comment made on an open Reddit forum (this could be considered trolling, but not cyberbullying, as explained above). The key difference between cyber-aggression and cyberbullying is that cyberbullying necessitates the interaction be intentional, personal, repeated, and with an intention to cause distress. Research has found that students who are cyberbullied have more negative consequences than those who are involved in cyber-aggression events [8]. This could be because of the fear engendered by the imbalance of power and

6 Social Media and Cyberbullying

There are several subtypes of cyberbullying, which could help one's understanding of how cyberbullying may be carried out. The most prominent forms cited both in research and colloquially among adolescents are as follows [9–11]:

- Exclusion
  - Exclusion is the act of leaving someone out deliberately, thereby stigmatizing them. Exclusion exists with traditional face-to-face bullying situations, but is also used in an online context. For example, a child might be excluded from a group invitation or special online group, while they see other friends being included, or left out of message threads or conversations that involve mutual friends.
- Harassment
  - Harassment is a broad term that encompasses many cyberbullying behaviors. It involves sending hurtful, offensive, or threatening messages to a target repeatedly.
- Denigration or Dissing
  - Denigration is when a cyberbully spreads untrue, hurtful, or damaging messages (either publicly or privately) about a target to others, in order to ruin their reputation or relationships with other people. In this situation, the cyberbully usually has a personal relationship with the victim.
- Masquerading or Impersonation
  - Masquerading is when the cyberbully creates a made-up profile or identity online with the sole purpose of targeting the victim. This could involve creating a fake online profile or social media account, with a new identity and photos to fool the cybervictim. A common example is the creation of a FINSTA or fake Instagram account to hide one's identity, or make it known to only a select group of individuals, in order to cyberbully anonymously.
- Outing/Doxing
  - Outing (also known as doxing) is when sensitive or personal information about a victim is revealed without their consent for the purpose of embarrassing or humiliating them. An example of this behavior is sharing photos of the victim or screenshotting personal messages with the victim and sharing them in a group message. The key element is the sharing of items without consent from the victim.
- Trickery
  - Trickery is similar to outing, with the addition of deception. In trickery, the bully will befriend the victim and give them a false sense of security. Once the bully has the target's trust, they abuse that trust and share private information the victim has shared to others without their consent.
- Trolling
  - Trolling is when a bully will intentionally upset a victim by posting inflammatory comments online. Trolling is not always a form of cyberbullying, but it can be when the comments are made with malicious intent to personally attack a target. If the bully does not have a relationship to their victim, or any ill intent, then it is considered trolling, but not cyberbullying.
- Flaming
  - Flaming is when a person sends angry, rude, or vulgar messages privately or publicly in a forum, or group. Flaming is similar to trolling, but flaming will usually be a more direct attack on a target.
- Cyberstalking
  - Cyberstalking is persistent, unwanted online monitoring or contact with a target. This may include surveilling a target, or obtaining personal information about a target's whereabouts. Cyberstalker conduct is often repetitive, invasive, and threatening. Cyberstalking is a criminal offense, and can result in a restraining order, probation, and even jail time for the perpetrator.
- Fraping
  - When a bully takes over another person's social networking account to post inappropriate content under their name. For example, a cyberbully posting racial or homophobic slurs through a cybervictim's account, and subsequently ruining their reputation.

Fig. 6.1 Cyberbullying subtypes

concern over repetition that is true only for cyberbullying and not for cyber-aggression [8]. As we are investigating cyberbullying and not cyber-aggressions at large, it is essential to recognize this distinction.

While numerous studies have focused on the outcomes of cyberbullying generally, less attention has been given to how and in what way cyberbullying via social media has impacted our youth. Social media is defined as "online communication networks that allow users to create their own content and engage in social interaction with both large and small audiences synchronously or asynchronously" [6]. Recent evidence suggests that social media plays a significant role in cyberbullying victimization and perpetration, with major impacts on well-being, which may be even more significant than cyberbullying that occurs via other modalities [12]. In this chapter, we will further explore cyberbullying and its definition, the prevalence of cyberbullying, and the consequences of cyberbullying. Special attention will be given to cyberbullying in the context of social media, and these insights will be embedded throughout the chapter.

Differentiating Cyberbullying from Traditional Bullying

Cyberbullying and traditional bullying are similar in various ways—they both involve aggressively ridiculing another individual, an imbalance of power wherein the perpetrator is more powerful, and a repetitive nature. There are studies to support a strong correlation between traditional and cyberbullying [13]. For example, a majority of cyberbullying perpetrators and victims are also bullying perpetrators and victims, respectively, and both types have a resulting psychological impact on all who are involved [13]. Like bullying, cyberbullying has an impact in the school environment; cyberbully events may either be triggered by issues at school or may result in academic difficulties. Cybervictims may identify a perpetrator as someone they know from school, as victims frequently know their perpetrator in "real life" [13]. Given these similarities, some argue that cyberbullying is simply bullying in another realm, with the primary difference being that cyberbullying takes place via an electronic format. As researchers have gained a better understanding of cyberbullying, however, several significant differentiating factors have been identified, barring cyberbullying from such a distilled definition.

Firstly, definitions of power imbalance do not clearly translate into a digital environment. Whereas with traditional bullying, an "imbalance of power" might refer to differences in physical strength or social status, cyberbullying may reflect differences in technology expertise or access to certain platforms [14]. Cyberbullies may also draw power from their ability to remain anonymous. Compared to traditional bullying, where incidents are isolated to face-to-face contact between children, cyberbullying allows for people to message, post, and create content anonymously. Tech-savvy teenagers can easily create fake social media accounts to harass others via posts, comments, and messages, without ever revealing their identity. The anonymity inherent in many cyberbullying situations may create a sense of powerlessness on the part of the victim, tipping the imbalance of power scale in the perpetrator's favor [7].

The potential threat of anonymity is compounded by the fact that cyberbullying can occur anywhere, and the aggressor does not have to see the victim's immediate reaction to their perpetration [15]. In this respect, teens are more likely to write or post content they wouldn't otherwise share face-to-face, because they don't realize the emotional harm they are causing. Reactions such as crying, yelling, or fighting back, which normally may lead aggressors to stop or regret their actions, are unseen online [7]. This distorted feedback, and underestimation of harm to a victim, may lead a cyberbully to be more ruthless and uncensored. It is often easier to be cruel using technology, because cyberbullying lacks this element of emotional reactivity [7].

In cyberbullying, there are also varying definitions for repetition. Unlike traditional bullying, where multiple offenses require multiple interactions, or multiple bullies, with cyberbullying a single offense can have a perpetual effect [5]. One cyberbully event can be multiplied one hundred times over if a message or a picture is shared with different individuals. These individuals may then further perpetuate the attack by forwarding messages to others, sharing harmful messages about the subject, or writing disparaging comments on a post. Due to online posting abilities, targets of cyberbullying are frequently harassed in front of larger audiences as compared to traditional bullying.

The pervasiveness of electronic bullying is also of particular concern, as cyberbullies can create posts defaming someone online at any time, meaning targets can experience this particular type of bullying even within their own home. This is in contrast to traditional bullying, which typically occurs in a more restricted, physical area [5]. Children's continuous access to the virtual world, where messages can be distributed quickly and to a broad audience, makes it more challenging to escape painful situations and find relief when being victimized [16]. Cyberbullying is also more easily disseminated, and the content communicated through online vectors is often permanent and public if not reported or removed. Even when removed from a site, content can remain on a person's phone via a screenshot or screen recording. While both traditional bullying and electronic bullying are detrimental to students, it is suspected that due to easier, faster, and more widespread transmission of cyberbullying, it might have an even more detrimental impact [17].

For authority figures, cyberbullying may be more difficult to recognize than traditional bullying, given the lack of face-to-face contact. Because teachers and parents may not overhear or see cyberbullying taking place as they may with traditional bullying, it may take more time to discover this type of bullying [4]. While caretakers are overall improving in terms of monitoring children's online activity, many adults don't have the technological skills (or time) to keep track of what is happening online [15]. Additionally, when cyberbullying is done anonymously, it may also be hard to identify the perpetrator, and even if the bully is identified, many adults find themselves unprepared to respond adequately [15]. The obscurity of cyberbullying presents new challenges for individuals, families, schools, professionals, researchers, and policymakers.

Unique Features of Cyberbullying via Social Media

Whereas adolescents used to spend time together in physical locations, socialization is increasingly happening in cyberspace, and subsequently, bullying has been taken from in-person to the cyberworld as well. In the early 2000s, the most popular place for youth to hang out was in chatrooms, and as a result, chatrooms were where most harassment took place. Today, with most adolescents drawn to social networking sites, there has been an increase in cyberbullying occurring through this modality.

Cyberbullying occurs across a variety of venues and mediums in cyberspace, and it shouldn't come as a surprise that it occurs most often where adolescents congregate online. In the early 2000s, the most popular place for youth to hang out was in chatrooms, and as a result, this is where most harassment took place. Today, with most youth drawn to social networking sites, there has been an increase in cyberbullying occurring through this modality.

Several authors have identified unique features of social media that may make cyberbullying victimization and perpetration more likely. Factors that may make social media a particularly appealing modality for cyberbullying include accessibility (e.g., a bully can reach a target at any place and anytime, with or without the presence of victim), information retrieval (e.g., finding out information about a target), editability (e.g., the bully can edit or delete a post and then deny cyberbullying ever occurred), and association (e.g., the bully can blame others for cyberbullying, and not be held accountable for actions) [6].

Other studies note that social media sites that allow for greater anonymity of posts increase likelihood for cyberbullying perpetration to occur compared to platforms where users are more identifiable (like Facebook, Instagram, and Snapchat). Anonymous social media sites, such as Yik Yak or Whisper, where users are allowed to post messages, photos, and videos anonymously, have long-standing controversy due to their inherent potential for cyberbullying. Due to widespread bullying and harassment, which occurred on the Yik Yak platform, many schools took action to have the app banned [18].

Another aspect of social media is the desire adolescents have to obtain likes and friends, or "go viral." The more followers one has or the more likes one has on a post, influences his or her popularity, and may be considered a status symbol or provide identity validation among adolescents. As youth work to achieve this goal, they may indiscriminately connect with others, which potentially exposes them to increased opportunities to be victimized [6]. In one longitudinal study on social media use, it was found that using social media was correlated with positive attitudes toward cyberbullying and increased likelihood of cyberbullying perpetration [6]. Risk factors for both cybervictims and cyberbullies in the context of social media will be further explored later in the chapter.

Prevalence of Cyberbullying, and its Challenges

There is no question that the use of smartphones, internet, social media, and overall electronic devices has increased exponentially over the last decade. According to the Pew Research Center, adolescents' access to smartphones has increased from 73% in 2015 to 95% in 2018 [19]. Simultaneously, adolescents report an increase in web activity, with 89% reporting they are online more than once a day and 45% reporting they are on the web "almost constantly." Among these teens who have access to smartphones and internet, social media use is pervasive, with 85% of

U.S. teens 13–17 years of age saying they spend time on YouTube, 72% on Instagram, 69% on Snapchat, 51% on Facebook, and 32% on Twitter [19]. When assessed by racial groups, White teens (41%) were more likely than Hispanic teens (29%) or Black teens (23%) to use Snapchat. Black teens (26%) were significantly more likely to use Facebook than White teens (7%) [19].

Anywhere from 10% to 70% of adolescents have reported cybervictimization, with the percentage increasing in recent years [20–23]. In 2018, the Pew Research Center reported that 59% of children aged 13–17 in the United States had experienced at least one of six types of harassing behaviors, which included offensive name-calling (42%), spreading of false rumors (32%), receiving explicit images they didn't ask for (25%), constant asking about their location, activities, and companions by someone other than a parent (21%), physical threats (16%), and having explicit images of them shared without their consent (7%) [24]. These statistics have become very worrisome to parents. In a survey of parents, 57% worry that their teen is involved in sending or receiving explicit images and 25% percent of parents mention that this concerns them significantly [24].

Studies regarding the prevalence of cyberbullying in the context of social media overall show that rates of cyberbullying events on these platforms are increasing [6]. In one study on U.S. college students, 18.2% of those sampled had experienced cyberbullying, and social media sites were one of the most common platforms in which these events occurred [14]. Similarly, another study found that 19% of college students reported cyberbullying victimization via social media and 46% witnessed cyberbullying on these sites [6]. This increasing prevalence has also been demonstrated on a global scale. In a study using a Canadian teens/young adult sample population, those who use social media were found to be 5.5 times more likely to experience cybervictimization than teens or young adults who did not use social media [25]. A large-scale study of 180,919 adolescents in 42 countries also found that social media use was positively correlated with both cyberbullying victimization and perpetration [26]. Instead of looking at global relationships between social media use and cybervictimization, other researchers have sought to understand how cyberbullying occurs on specific social media platforms. For example, in a study of tweets that specifically referred to a cyberbullying situation, 60% out of 38,197 tweets were related to a specific cyberbullying event [27].

While there are many studies on the prevalence of cyberbullying, there is debate over the accuracy of study findings as prevalence rates of cyberbullying are highly variable across studies. For example, in a review article published in the Journal of Adolescent Health regarding the prevalence among U.S. middle- and high-school-aged adolescents, which distinguished high-quality studies from poor quality in their systemic findings, there was a wide range of study results for the prevalence of cyberbullying, even among studies that were considered high-quality results [22]. The study found that the prevalence of cyberbullying victimization and perpetration was heavily affected by the period of time measured (e.g., whether cyberbullying occurred in the last month, year, or lifetime) [22]. When data was stratified based on time period, the results across studies were highly inconsistent. It was found that the prevalence of cybervictimization in the last one month was 5.9% to 29.4% (3 studies), in the last year was 4.3–40.6% (6 studies), and "ever" was 23% (1 study) [22].

For cyberbullying perpetration, the prevalence in the last one month was 4.9–21.8% (2 studies), and in the last year was 15–41% (3 studies) [22]. In all, the systematic review found the prevalence of cyberbullying victimization ranged from 3% to 72%, while perpetration ranged from 1% to 41% [22]. Seemingly, time intervals embedded in the study design can strongly influence prevalence outcomes.

Several other factors likely contribute to inconsistencies in studies on cyberbullying prevalence, including varying definitions used for "cyberbullying," the ages of participants, how youth are recruited for the study (online vs. at school), and the lack of valid and reliable questionnaires used to query research participants, and inconsistencies in the analysis of responses [14]. A primary difficulty with defining cyberbullying is how the word and definition is translated depending on one's country, language, and culture. The word "cyberbullying" has a different meaning and definition depending on the country, language, and culture. In some countries, cyberbullying may include any form of cyber-harassment, which makes it difficult to gain a comprehensive understanding of prevalence changes in a global scale. Additionally, studies have a wide range in how they defined repeatedness, which is embedded in the cyberbullying definition in this chapter. In some studies, even one instance of intentional cyber-harmfulness was considered cyberbullying, as this one act could arguably be seen multiple times by multiple people. Others only included cyberbullying experiences that occurred multiple times.

There are also a range of ways in which studies have chosen to incorporate the concept of "cyberbullying" within the study design, even when studying the same country and culture. Many studies have utilized a measure of cyberbullying that does not provide a definition for cyberbullying or use the word "bully" in order to avoid the issue of labeling students as "bullies" or "victims," or to be inclusive of participants whose experiences differ from the definition [7]. While it's helpful to capture more affected youth, these varying definitions may also contribute to difficulty in determining the true prevalence of cyberbullying. A study found that 72% of youth had been involved in cyberbullying victimization; however, the term cyberbullying was not specifically used in their study design [28]. Instead, participants were asked if they had experienced "mean things" online, which was defined as "anything that someone else does that upsets or offends someone" [28]. Conceivably, the wording used in this study would result in higher prevalence rates for cyberbullying.

When comparing studies which used broad questions regarding whether participants had ever been a victim or perpetrator of cyberbullying versus had they ever been cyberbullied via a number of different avenues, there was the opposite effect on prevalence rates. Surprisingly, when participants were asked a single, broad question of whether they have encountered cyberbullying, the prevalence rate decreased dramatically compared to when asked specific questions about cyberbullying and the particular avenue through which it occurred [14]. Overall, global single item questions such as "Have you been cyberbullied?" tend to lead to fewer responses compared to behavioral questions such as "Have you ever been sent a mean text message?" mainly because students do not consider some of the specific behaviors to be bullying [8].

Beyond these challenges, rapidly changing technologies and online trends also contribute to variability in study results, as changing modalities for cyberbullying may influence study outcomes. In 2007, instant messaging was found to be the most frequently used avenue for cyberbullying reported by both victims and perpetrators [16]. Just 2 years later, chat rooms were observed to be the most common method of peer-to-peer communication and cyberbullying among middle- and high-school students [16]. Today, social media has emerged as the most common modality for cyberbullying victimization and perpetration [29]. It is likely that the most pervasive avenues for cyberbullying today will be different in a decade, which makes it difficult to reliably gain insights from studies.

Given the above variance in cyberbullying studies, it would be helpful to have more research that is longitudinal or experimental in nature, with consistent study designs inclusive of varying cultures, and more precise definitions for cyberbullying. In spite of these difficulties, the fact remains that cyberbullying is a serious problem confronting adolescents today, requiring further research to better understand its nature and how it may impact our youth.

Cyberbullying Victimization and Perpetration Risk Factors

Recognizing the circumstances and mindsets that place children at higher risk of becoming cyberbullies can help us gather a deeper understanding about the origin and execution of cyberbullying. The various individual characteristics, attitudes, desires, personalities, and motives of a cyberperpetrator, and likewise those of a cybervictim, largely contribute to the course of a cyberbullying interaction and how it will be handled. Risk factors for cyberbullying events (as either a victim or a perpetrator) can generally be categorized into two broad categories—personal factors and situational factors [14]. Personal factors refer to individual characteristics, including age, gender, race, socioeconomic status, online behavior, personality traits, and past experiences of victimization, while situational factors refer to interpersonal relationships, provocation and perceived support, parental involvement and school support [7]. Protective factors against cyberbullying include empathy, emotional intelligence, good parent-child relationship, and school climate.

Cyberbullying Victimization Risk

In a meta-analysis studying cyberbullying risk factors in 2021, the most consistent personal factors contributing to cybervictimization included female gender, prior history of mental health problems (such as depression, eating disorders, borderline personality disorder, insomnia, and suicidal ideation), and increased time spent on the internet [30]. In terms of situational risk factors for cybervictimization, studies have demonstrated risk may increase with parental abuse, parental neglect, family dysfunction, inadequate monitoring, and parents' inconsistency in mediation and communication [30]. Additionally, studies showed geographical factors contributed to risk, and that adolescents who live in city locations may be more at risk for victimization compared to those in suburban areas [30].

There are also individual factors that may impact risk for cybervictimization in the context of social media specifically, including low agreeableness, high extraversion and openness to experience, low emotional stability and LGBTQ+ status [6]. A few additional factors include self-disclosure, disposition, and emotional stability [31]. Social status can impact cyberbullying risk. Having fewer or weak friendships within a victims' social network is negatively correlated with social status [32]. Adolescents perceived as "low status" by their peers (e.g. a large amount of unbalanced and weak friendships within one's network of online connections) were found to be at higher risk for perpetration [31, 32]. Research also found these victims were less likely to be defended by peers and the perpetrators who antagonized them were less likely to be viewed negatively [31].

How users engage on social media may also intentionally or unintentionally invite perpetration [31]. Online risky conduct, such as posting inappropriate, profane or hurtful comments led to a greater risk of victimhood [33]. Other research on adolescent online activity have found that problematic social media use, social media addiction, indiscreet posting, and number of followers were all linked to increased risk of cyberbullying victimization [34]. These behaviors also impact how bystanders might react. Research has shown that bystanders become less empathetic and less motivated to intervene or defend a victim if the victim was perceived to have disclosed indiscreet information on social media [35].

There is also evidence that social media use may not increase vulnerability to cybervictimization. In a longitudinal study of German youth, social media was not found to predict future cyberbullying or cybervictimization. However, cyberbullying involvement was predictive of future social media use [36]. It is proposed that the victims of cyberbullying are subsequently using social media to retaliate against the individuals who bullied them [36]. These authors speculate that perhaps cyberbullying intervention programs should focus on the way adolescents use social media, rather than the frequency of use [36].

Cyberbullying Perpetration Risk

There have been several predictive factors found to increase one's risk of engaging in cyberbullying. A leading personal factor that tends to increase risk of initiating cyberbullying via social media includes presence of normative thinking, peer pressure, and involvement in a peer group where aggressive behavior is normalized [37]. As adolescents begin to develop a sense of identity and independence, the most important relationships in their lives shift from family towards peers. If one's peers have normalized cyberbullying behavior, this will greatly influence an adolescent's view of cyberbullying perpetration, even if it contradicts their previously existing moral beliefs [37].

In social media specific studies, researchers found dark-side personality traits (such as sadism and narcissism), low-self-esteem, depressive symptoms, low empathy, moral disengagement, and childhood emotional trauma all contributed to an elevated risk of cyberbully perpetration [6]. Other personal factors found to increase risk of cyberbullying perpetration include hyperactivity and inattention difficulties, behavior problems, school-related problems, and risky behaviors on the internet (e.g. posting personal information, using a web camera, and harassment of others online) [38]. Studies have also consistently shown that individuals who have previously experienced either cyberbullying or traditional bullying as a victim tended to be at higher risk for becoming cyberbullying perpetrators (but not face-to-face aggressors). This indicates a possible cyclical nature to cyberbullying, as the experience of cybervictimization may provoke one to engage in cyberbullying perpetration themselves [7]. The association between cyberbullying and technology usage also comes into play here, as perpetrators may learn bullying behaviors through bullying-related events they have observed on the internet [31].

When considering situational factors that increase risk for cyberbullying perpetration, weaker familial emotional bonds, school detachment, as well as conflictual teacher-student relationships, are prominent risks. Parenting styles may also contribute to risk. This includes parents who are considered either overcontrolling with an authoritarian parenting style, or, on the other end of the spectrum, parents who are more permissive with less involvement in online behavior and poor rule setting [39]. Similar to cybervictim geographical risk factors, studies have found that adolescents who reside in cities are more likely to be cyberbully perpetrators than those living in more rural areas [30]. Growing up in a low-income household was positively correlated with likelihood of perpetration [37]. It is posed that students from low-income backgrounds are more likely to engage in cyberbullying behavior, because their social development and peer interactions may be limited if they are not able to participate in certain activities due to a payment gap [37].

Cyberbullying Demographics and Its Challenges

While many studies have focused on risks for cyberbullying victimization and perpetration, there is often conflicting evidence found in studies, especially regarding demographic risk factors. This section will further explore the conflicting outcomes of research on age, gender, and being part of a minority group in the context of cyberbullying.

Age

Regarding cyberbullying demographics based on age, there are variable study results. However, most studies show that the risk for cybervictimization increases as children approach their adolescent years [40, 41], reaching its highest prevalence around age 15. For cyberbullying perpetrators, it is also believed that older teenagers, especially those older than 15, are at greater risk [30]. Despite these results, this age demographic is known to be rapidly changing as children are beginning to have access to smartphones and the internet at an earlier age [42]. In a recent study, children as young as elementary school are now reporting being the victim of cyberbullying, and this is directly linked to their exposure of the internet at an earlier age [30]. Up to 85% of preteens are reported to be using web-based messaging, and this access substantially increases children's opportunities for cybervictimization [43].

In social media specific studies, several studies found that cyberbullying tends to occur in similar age groups and the frequency of cyberbullying tends to increase with age [12]. There was also evidence that younger children are more vulnerable to psychological distress as a result of cyberbullying compared to older adolescents. However, there was also conflicting evidence, with several studies showing that age had no impact on cyberbullying or exposure to cyberbullying [12]. More recent studies have shown that girls aged between 12 and 15 years are more likely to be victims of cyberbullying and were more likely to show problematic social media use than boys [44].

Gender

Studies are conflicting in regards to how gender factors into cyberbullying. Many studies have speculated that cybervictimization tends to be higher in girls than in boys [30, 45–49], and other studies indicating results are mixed and there is no unanimity [50, 51]. Similarly, studies on gender differences of cyberbully perpetrators are also inconsistent, with many studies showing there is no statistically significant difference between girls and boys in rates of cyberbullying perpetration or victimization [2, 40, 52–54]. Still, other research found boys are more likely than girls to perpetrate cyberbullying, but found that either there are no gender differences in terms of victimization [47] or that girls were more likely to be victimized [55]. One group of investigators suggest that gender differences depend on the venue by which the cyberbullying occurs; for example, girls seem to be targeted via e-mail more frequently than boys [52], whereas boys are more often bullied through text messaging [2, 28, 53].

This is in contrast to studies on traditional bullying, which has more consistently shown that male adolescents are more likely to engage in physical and verbal bullying, and girls less so [61]. In traditional bullying research, female adolescents have been found to be relatively more likely to engage in relational bullying (e.g. social exclusion) and indirect forms of bullying (not face-to-face, rumor spreading). This might lead one to theoretically presume girls are more likely to engage in cyberbullying (both as a victim and perpetrator), given its common indirect nature, however, this has not been consistently found in the literature.

In a review of cyberbullying within the context of social media [12] conflictual evidence was found regarding gender differences. Most studies in the review seemed to find that girls were more likely to be cybervictims than boys [12]. Boys were more likely than girls to be cyberbully perpetrators, engage in direct bullying, and tended to be more repetitive in their cyberbullying [12]. Two studies in the review, however, found there was no difference between sexes in terms of likelihood of cybervictimization [2, 56]. An investigation of cybervictimization via Facebook in 2016 found that certain studied individual characteristics such as low agreeableness and more time spent on Facebook were predictive of male cybervictimization, whereas for females none of the variables studied predicted involvement in cyberbullying [57].

Minority Youth

Despite many studies evaluating the relationship between ethnicity and cyberbullying behavior, exactly how and if ethnicity has a conclusive impact on cyberbullying activity remains unclear. A United States meta-analysis of over 100 studies on peer victimization discovered that on average, Caucasian youth are subject to more peer victimization than ethnic minority youth [49, 58]. Similarly, in a multiethnic study of cyberbullying and mental health, Caucasians were found to have the highest frequency of cybervictimization experiences [49, 59]. In a literature review looking at cyberbullying through the lens of race and ethnicity [60], significant inconsistencies were found in the rate of victimization by race across studies (Black: 4% to 17%; Hispanic: 6% to 13%; White: 18% to 30%); perpetration (Black: 7% to 11%; Hispanic: 16% to 18%; White: 4% to 42%). Other researches analyzing cyberbullying among various ethnic groups have also found variability [59, 61]. Research on racial differences in the experience of cyberbullying found that responses between black and white participants did not differ markedly, further complicating the picture of how race may factor into the cyberbullying experience [29].

According to a review on cyberbullying in the context of social media, seven studies which evaluated the relationship between ethnicity and cyberbullying behavior were cited [12]. One study on Canadian youth between age 11 and 15 found that 10–20% reported that they had occasionally experienced cyberbullying related to race [62]. One study in the United States found that white and Hispanic adolescents were more likely to be involved in cyberbullying, which conflicted with a different study in the United States where white (72%) and Hispanic (78%) youth reported to feel others were mainly kind to them online, compared to black youth (56%). Another study explored the differences between cyberbullying among Native Hawaiian, white, Filipino and Samoan individuals, and found prevalence of cyberbullying ranged from 48.8% (Samoan) to 62.2% (white). Three other studies referenced in the review conversely showed there was no effect of ethnicity on cyberbullying behavior [63].

Specific to sexual and gender minority youth, there is a dearth of research on the experiences of LGBTQ youth and cyberbullying, despite research showing that sexual minorities are one of the most vulnerable populations to this type of bullying [51, 64]. A systematic literature review [64] found a more direct correlation between cybervictimization and adverse effects for sexual minority and gender-expansive adolescents than for their heterosexual and cisgender counterparts. These children experience cyberbullying in the form of being "outed," exposed, and harassed due to their sexual and gender identity, and social media is one of the prevalent platforms on which this occurs [64]. Findings illustrated that the rate of cyberbullying among LGBTQ youth is between 10.5% and 71.3%. LGBTQ youth who have been victims of cyberbullying have confronted various negative outcomes, including psychological and emotional disturbances (such as suicidal ideation and attempts, depression, and lower self-esteem), behavioral issues (such as physical aggression, problematic body images, and social isolation), and poorer academic performances (such as lower GPAs) [64].

Specific to sexual and gender minority youth, there is a dearth of research on the experiences of LGBTQ youth and cyberbullying, despite research showing that sexual minorities are one of the most vulnerable populations to this type of bullying [51, 64]. A more direct correlation between cybervictimization and adverse effects for sexual minority and gender-expansive adolescents than for their heterosexual and cisgender counterparts has been found [64]. These children experience cyberbullying in the form of being "outed," exposed, and harassed due to their sexual and gender identity, and social media is one of the prevalent platforms on which this occurs [64]. Findings illustrated that the rate of cyberbullying among LGBTQ youth is between 10.5% and 71.3%. LGDTQ youth who have been victims of cyberbullying have confronted various negative outcomes, including psychological and emotional disturbances (such as suicidal ideation and attempts, depression, and lower self-esteem), behavioral issues (such as physical aggression, problematic body images, and social isolation), and poorer academic performances (such as lower GPAs).

Mental Health Impact of Cyberbullying

Mental health effects of cyberbullying are crucial to understand, as outcomes are related to suicide and depression. Since the early 2000s, studies have found cyberbullying to be associated with negative feelings, such as embarrassment, worry, fear, depression, or loneliness [38]. Studies examining mental health effects of cyberbullying victimization have correlated the experience with low self-esteem, depression, anxiety, family problems, academic difficulties, school violence, suicidal thoughts, and self-injurious behaviors [12]. Most of the studies focusing on these harmful effects, however, had broad and varying definitions for cyberbullying. Even fewer studies have focused on cyberbullying in the context of social media, which, given its pervasiveness in society and subsequent impact on youth, deserves specialized attention.

Researchers have speculated that cyberbullying via social media is more damaging than cyberbullying through other online communication methods, especially if posts are public or easily seen by peers [4]. In social media specific studies, cybervictims have reported a multitude of effects, including becoming more withdrawn, losing confidence and self-esteem, and developing a general sense of uneasiness after a cyberbullying event [12]. Additionally, relationships have been shown to be negatively impacted, especially those with family members, friends, and partners. Other negative outcomes for those involved in cyberbullying via social media include increased levels of psychological distress and physical complaints [65],

6 Social Media and Cyberbullying

reduced life satisfaction [66], and suicidal ideation and attempts [25]. Several studies showed levels of depression and anxiety significantly increase with exposure to cyberbullying [12]. It may also increase the likelihood of engaging in risky behaviors including alcohol and substance use.

Other research has shown that enduring cyberbullying, while using social media, can impact the victims' perception of interpersonal relationships and negatively impact their opinions about broader organizations, including their outlook on school. For example, a study on Israeli students who had experienced cyberbullying in a Whatsapp classroom group felt less of a sense of belonging among their peers and general negative feelings toward their school's social culture [67].

The outcomes experienced may depend, in part, on the response offered by the cyberbullying victims. For example, in a study on college students and cyberbullying, cybervictims reported they either blocked or confronted the bully or stayed off social media to avoid further perpetration [14]. The negative consequences of experiencing cyberbullying via social media may also depend on the number of stressors involved. The consequences of online harassment is directly correlated with the number of stress factors, such as the presence of multiple perpetrators, repetition, and contact with the cyberbully (or cyberbullies) offline [68].

Fewer studies have looked at the well-being of cyberbullying perpetrators on social media [6]. Cyberbullies often expressed various physical health complaints, including headaches and dizziness [65]. A link has been found between cyberbullying perpetration and a lower sense of belonging, as well as an increased likelihood of depression secondary to problematic social media use [69]. Despite this evidence, other research has found no association between well-being and cyberbullying behaviors [6]. For example, cyberbullying perpetrators did not experience unique levels of anxiety or self-perceptions of mattering [70]. This discordance across studies highlights a need for additional research that explores the relationship between cyberbullying perpetration on social media and well-being [6].

Cyberbullying Protective Factors

Some factors may make it less likely for individuals to engage in cyberbullying perpetration. One of the major concerns with cyberbullying via social media is the ability to post anonymously and recklessly, without fear of retribution from social media networking sites. Youth with higher awareness and perceived ability to control information shared on social media were less likely to become victims. It seems adolescents may benefit from education on how to make social media accounts more private and secure [71].

On a personal level, studies have found that high emotional intelligence, an ability to self-regulate emotions, and empathy, were associated with lower rates of cyberbullying [30]. Emotional self-efficacy served as a mediator between cyberbullying victimization and self-esteem, perceived social support, and subjective sense of well-being [72]. Less rumination over cyberbullying event with improved sense of self-esteem and life satisfaction [73].

At a situational level, perceived presence of social support has also shown to have a positive role on well-being and reduce vulnerability to the negative effects of cyberbullying [39]. The parent role is also critical, as open communication and strong parent-child relationships have been shown to reduce the likelihood of cyberbullying [39]. Having a supportive high-school environment has also been shown to be protective, especially if the school works synergistically with parents to optimize support for youth [39].

Tips for Parents

The constantly evolving technological landscape poses added challenges to parenting in the digital era, which requires a balance between allowing children to explore and learn independently, while maintaining an appropriate level of parental supervision and ensuring their safety. This delicate and ever-shifting balance can only be achieved if parents teach children at a young age to use those vast digital resources responsibly, while giving them a sense of trust and support in navigating the complex world of digital communications.

The best way of preventing cyberbullying is knowing what children are doing online, what websites they are visiting, who they are connecting with, and how to set up age-appropriate safety features. Having open and honest conversations with children, and allowing them a nonjudgmental and safe setting for expressing their concerns, is ultimately the best means of helping prevent cyberbullying. Through those ongoing and regular conversations with children, parents might be able to gauge their child's ability to recognize the signs of cyberbullying, whether it is happening to the child or if they are acting as a perpetrator of bullying. It is crucial to help them recognize forms of cyberbullying, whether they are being bullied, bullying others, or witnessing bullying [4].

Parents should also educate themselves on what's an appropriate time to give a child their first cell phone or tablet, how to set limits on screen time, and how to understand signs of unhealthy use of screen time and online content. Once the child has become an active participant in social media, it is important for parents to stay involved and continue to engage their children in an open dialogue, as the digital world continues to grow and change with new apps and new platforms.

Below are a few links for resources on prevention of cyberbullying:
https://www.stopbullying.gov/
https://www.cdc.gov/
https://www.nctsn.org/
https://www.connectsafely.org/cyberbullying/
https://www.parents.com/kids/problems/bullying/18-tips-to-stop-cyberbullying/
https://childmind.org/article/help-kids-deal-cyberbullying/
https://centerforparentingeducation.org/library-of-articles/handling-bullying-issues/cyber-bullying-what-parents-can-do-about-it/
https://www.pta.org/home/family-resources/safety/Digital-Safety/Parents-Can-Prevent-Cyberbullying

https://www.familyzone.com/anz/families/blog/cyberbullying-practical-tips-for-parents

https://nij.ojp.gov/- The National Institute of Justice Office of Justice Program

Below are some noteworthy points and recommendations summarized from the above cited resources regarding prevention of cyberbullying.

Warning Signs that a Child is Being Cyberbullied or is Cyberbullying Others are:

- Becoming upset, sad, or angry during or after using the internet or their phone.
- Being very secretive or protective of their online activities, hiding their screen or switching screens when someone walks in.
- Withdrawing from their family, friends, and activities they previously enjoyed.
- Avoiding school; becoming depressed or anxious, or losing interest in previously enjoyed social gatherings.
- Deteriorating grades at school and/or "acting out" at home; changes in mood, behavior, sleep, or appetite.
- Complaining of aches and pains and various illnesses in order to stay home from school or to avoid social gatherings.
- Increasing or decreasing use of their electronic devices. Unusual behavior, such as shutting down their social medical accounts or opening new ones.
- Being nervous or jumpy when getting a message, text, or email and avoiding discussions about computer or phone activities.

Before Children Start Using Internet

Ideally preventing cyberbullying starts long before a child is actively using the internet and particularly social media. Parents establish trust from a very young age by having regular honest conversations with their children, continuously teaching them appropriate values and expectations, and, most importantly—listening to their children. Listening is likely the most critical tool in preventing unhealthy uses of technology, including cyberbullying.

When such a trusting dialog exists, children are more likely to share their digital experiences and discuss any unpleasant interactions, giving the parents ample opportunities to address any potential risks and employ proper corrective actions when needed. When children feel that their parents are looking out for their safety, they are more likely to participate in an open dialogue and to hear their parents' perspective.

Once They Start Using the Internet

It is important for parents to familiarize themselves with popular forms of social media and to know which one of them is being preferentially used by their child. The moment parents joined Facebook and became proficient in navigating its use, kids switched to Instagram and "Snapchat, and Facebook was no longer "cool" among young people. Now children often text, or use gaming platforms where they connect live while playing video games via various consoles. Parents should ask questions and stay up-to-date with their children's online activities. Specifically, parents should ask their children to "add" and "friend" and teach them how to use the platform. Younger children like having their parents and siblings involved and interested, and they like to share and "teach" about social media. Conversely, teenagers may become more secretive as they get older. Ultimately, kids who have their parent's trust are more likely to share and express their concerns when faced with unwanted interactions online.

Although it is impossible to know everything about children's online activities, here are some suggestions for parents on preventing unhealthy digital behaviors as summarized from various websites listed above:

- If possible, try to keep the computer in a common area, and not children's bedrooms.
- Have the privacy settings on all electronic devices allowing to monitor a teen's social media use, apps, and browsing history. Review or regularly re-set your child's phone location and privacy settings.
- Set clear expectations about digital behavior and online reputation (such as posting hateful speech or comments, sexting, and sharing naked photos of themselves or others, discuss potential legal problems that might arise from such behaviors).
- Become familiar with media platforms like Facebook, Instagram, and Twitter. Ask your children if they will show you their profile pages.
- Ask to follow or friend your child on their social media sites or have another reliable adult do so. Have your child's user names and passwords for email and social media.
- Learn about popular apps and identify which ones are appropriate for your child (content and age-wise).
- Establish rules and set limits on how much time a child can spend online or on their devices. Ask your children to take part in establishing the rules; then, they'll be more likely to follow them
- Maintain the trusting and open relationship and talk to children regularly, encourage them to come to you for help if they had any concerning interactions online. Continue to listen attentively, in a supportive and nonjudgmental manner.

What to Do When Cyberbullying Happens?

If a child's behavior is suggestive of possible involvement in cyberbullying, parents should attend to the situation immediately but carefully. As stated above, there are warning signs that children display when engaged in cyberbullying, whether as victims or as perpetrators. Below are some suggestions and recommendations for parents, summarized from various sources:

6 Social Media and Cyberbullying

- Identify the warning signs (such as changes in mood or behavior) and explore if these behaviors are related to their online activities.
- Ask direct questions to find out what is happening, and listen attentively in a nonjudgmental manner to figure out how it started and who is involved.
- A child who is bullied should not be blamed, so try not to overreact by disciplining your child (e.g., taking away their devices, limiting their screen time etc.). It's helpful to be supportive of them, and ensure that the child is willing to work together on resolving the situation and finding a solution.
- Remember that parents who tend to react harshly and negatively by taking away their cell phones/tablets/consoles and barring internet use can damage trust and may be left unaware of cyberbullying.
- However, try not to shrug off or minimize their suffering by telling them to "ignore it" or "just deal with it." The harm from bullying can leave lifelong consequences.
- Instruct your children not to respond to any threats or unpleasant comments online, but also keep a record of those messages (e.g., take screenshots, or print out those messages). You will need the messages to verify and prove that there is cyberbullying. Data shows that bullying is a repeated behavior, so keeping records helps to fight such behavior.
- **If cyberbullying involves school, report it to the school. Parents can also contact the social media platforms directly** to report the offense.
- **Find support for your child from peers, mentors, and school counselors**, who can intervene to positively impact a situation in various positive ways. Sometimes, more professional help is needed (e.g., to speak to a mental health professional).
- In cases of a physical threats or illegal behavior (e.g., involving sex trafficking, drugs, weapons, etc.), report it to law enforcement agencies.

What to Do When a Child is a Witness of Cyberbullying

Talking to children about safe behavior online should be an ongoing education that helps them constantly learn and identify risks and threats, as well as consistently practice healthy ways of responding to potentially harmful situations. Kids with strong values and robust self-esteem are less likely to bully others, and more likely to both have a healthy response to bullying and to be a positive role model for others.

Here are some recommendations for parents, whose kids might be bystanders of cyberbullying and need some encouragement:

- Encourage children not to engage in cyberbullying by first recognizing it when it happens and second by not encouraging it. For example—ask children not to "like," share, or comment on posts about someone that are harmful. Refusing to engage may curb the potential harm to others and to themselves.
- Encourage a child who feels strongly that they must react to a post that they should respond in a calm and constructive way. Negative reactions can make a

potentially harmful situation worse and bring about retaliation. Encourage children to take a break from posting and take time to cool down and reassess the situation when calm.

Most of the major social medial platforms have created portals for parents where they can find more information on rules and restrictions that apply to minors. This is part of platform efforts to establish partnership with parents for safer use of social media by children. Knowledge of those rules is important in helping prevent and manage cyberbullying.

Multiple Choice Questions
1. What does the term "fraping" refer to?
   A. When personal information about someone else is revealed on the internet without their consent
   B. When a bully takes over another person's internet profile and posts inappropriate content under their name
   C. When a bully makes a fake internet profile for the sole purpose to harass another person
   Correct Answer: B
2. What personal factors have been found to contribute to cybervictimization:
   A. Having many internet followers and physical attractiveness
   B. Male gender, political interests, and high-grade point average
   C. Female gender, history of mental health issues, increased time spent on the internet
   Correct Answer: C
3. What is recommended that a parent do when they find out their child is a victim of cyberbullying?
   A. Ask direct nonjudgmental questions of the child to better understand the situation and who is involved
   B. Do nothing and pretend they are not aware so that their child can learn to problem solve independently
   C. Inform both the school board and the local police
   Correct Answer: A

References

1. John A, et al. Self-harm, suicidal behaviours, and cyberbullying in children and young people: systematic review. J Med Internet Res. 2018;20(4):e129.
2. Smith PK, et al. Cyberbullying: its nature and impact in secondary school pupils. J Child Psychol Psychiatry. 2008;49(4):376–85.
3. Triantafyllopoulou P, Clark-Hughes C, Langdon PE. Social media and cyber-bullying in autistic adults. J Autism Dev Disord. 2021:1–9.
4. What is cyberbullying. Stopbullying.gov [cited 2022 3/16/22]. www.stopbullying.gov/cyberbullying/index.html.
5. Anaraky RG, et al. The dark side of social media: what makes some users more vulnerable than others? In Conference companion publication of the 2019 on computer supported

6 Social Media and Cyberbullying

cooperative work and social computing. 2019, Association for Computing Machinery: Austin, TX, USA. p. 185–189.

6. Giumetti GW, Kowalski RM. Cyberbullying via social media and well-being. Curr Opin Psychol. 2022;45:101314.
7. Kowalski RM, et al. Bullying in the digital age: a critical review and meta-analysis of cyberbullying research among youth. Psychol Bull. 2014;140(4):1073–137.
8. Campbell M, Bauman S. Reducing cyberbullying in schools: international evidence-based best practices; 2018.
9. Watts LK, Velasquez B, Behrens PI. Cyberbullying in higher education: a literature review. Comput Human Behav. 2017;69:268–74.
10. Peled Y. Cyberbullying and its influence on academic, social, and emotional development of undergraduate students. Heliyon. 2019;5(3):e01393.
11. 10 forms of cyberbullying. Kids Safety 2015. https://kids.kaspersky.com/10-forms-of-cyberbullying/.
12. Hamm MP, et al. Prevalence and effect of cyberbullying on children and young people: a scoping review of social media studies. JAMA Pediatr. 2015;169(8):770–7.
13. Englander E, et al. Defining cyberbullying. Pediatrics. 2017;140(Suppl 2):S148–s151.
14. Whittaker E, Kowalski RM. Cyberbullying via social media. J School Violence. 2015;14(1):11–29.
15. Hinduja SP, et al. Cyberbullying identification, prevention, and response. Cyberbullying Research Center; 2021. Cyberbullying.org.
16. Kowalski RM, Limber SP. Electronic bullying among middle school students. J Adolesc Health. 2007;41(6 Suppl 1):S22–30.
17. Nikolaou D. Does cyberbullying impact youth suicidal behaviors? J Health Econ. 2017;56:30–46.
18. Clair N.R.a.S.S., Yik Yak app disabled in Chicago amid principals' worries; 2014.
19. Anderson M, Teens JJ. Social media and technology 2018. Pew Research Center; 2018. https://www.pewresearch.org/internet/2018/05/31/teens-social-media-technology-2018/
20. Kutok ER, et al. A cyberbullying media-based prevention intervention for adolescents on instagram: pilot randomized controlled trial. JMIR Ment Health. 2021;8(9):e26029.
21. Aboujaoude E, et al. Cyberbullying: review of an old problem gone viral. J Adolesc Health. 2015;57(1):10–8.
22. Selkie EM, Fales JL, Moreno MA. Cyberbullying prevalence among US middle and high school-aged adolescents: a systematic review and quality assessment. J Adolesc Health. 2016;58(2):125–33.
23. Hellstrand K, et al. Prevalence of cyberbullying in patients presenting to the pediatric emergency department. Pediatr Emerg Care. 2021;37(6):e334–8.
24. Andrew M, Jiang J. Social media and technology 2018. Pew Research Center; 2019. [cited 2022]. https://www.pewresearch.org/internet/2018/05/31/teens-social-media-technology-2018/.
25. Sampasa-Kanyinga H, Hamilton HA. Use of social networking sites and risk of cyberbullying victimization: a population-level study of adolescents. Cyberpsychol Behav Soc Netw. 2015;18(12):704–10.
26. Craig W, et al. Social media use and cyber-bullying: a cross-national analysis of young people in 42 countries. J Adolesc Health. 2020;66(6s):S100–s108.
27. McHugh MC, Saperstein SL, Gold RS. OMG U #Cyberbully! an exploration of public discourse about cyberbullying on twitter. Health Educ Behav. 2019;46(1):97–105.
28. Juvonen J, Gross EF. Extending the school grounds?--Bullying experiences in cyberspace. J Sch Health. 2008;78(9):496–505.
29. Kowalski RM, et al. Racial differences in cyberbullying from the perspective of victims and perpetrators. Am J Orthopsychiatry. 2020;90(5):644–52.
30. Zhu C, et al. Cyberbullying among adolescents and children: a comprehensive review of the global situation, risk factors, and preventive measures. Front Public Health. 2021;9:634909.
31. Chan TKH, Cheung CMK, Lee ZWY. Cyberbullying on social networking sites: a literature review and future research directions. Information Management. 2021;58(2):103411.

32. Wegge D, et al. The strong, the weak, and the unbalanced: the link between tie strength and cyberaggression on a social network site. Social Sci Comput Rev. 2015;33(3):315–42.
33. Peluchette JV, et al. Cyberbullying victimization: do victims' personality and risky social network behaviors contribute to the problem? Comput Human Behav. 2015;52:424–35.
34. Boer M, et al. Social media use intensity, social media use problems, and mental health among adolescents: investigating directionality and mediating processes. Comput Human Behav. 2021;116:106645.
35. Schacter HL, Greenberg S, Juvonen J. Who's to blame?: The effects of victim disclosure on bystander reactions to cyberbullying. Comput Human Behav. 2016;57:115–21.
36. Müller CR, et al. Does media use lead to cyberbullying or vice versa? Testing longitudinal associations using a latent cross-lagged panel design. Comput Human Behav. 2018;81:93–101.
37. Ademiluyi A, Li C, Park A. Implications and preventions of cyberbullying and social exclusion in social media: systematic review. JMIR Form Res. 2022;6(1):e30286.
38. Hoge E, Bickham D, Cantor J. Digital media, anxiety, and depression in children. Pediatrics. 2017;140(Suppl 2):S76 o80.
39. Marengo N, et al. Cyberbullying and problematic social media use: an insight into the positive role of social support in adolescents-data from the Health Behaviour in School-aged Children study in Italy. Public Health. 2021;199:46–50.
40. Fisher BW, Gardella JH, Teurbe-Tolon AR. Peer cybervictimization among adolescents and the associated internalizing and externalizing problems: a meta-analysis. J Youth Adolesc. 2016;45(9):1727–43.
41. Williams KR, Guerra NG. Prevalence and predictors of internet bullying. J Adolesc Health. 2007;41(6 Suppl 1):S14–21.
42. Machimbarrena JM, et al. Internet risks: an overview of victimization in cyberbullying, cyber dating abuse, sexting, online grooming and problematic internet use. Int J Environ Res Public Health. 2018;15(11)
43. Peng Z, et al. Associations between Chinese adolescents subjected to traditional and cyber bullying and suicidal ideation, self-harm and suicide attempts. BMC Psychiatry. 2019;19(1):324.
44. Morin HK, Bradshaw CP, Kush JM. Adjustment outcomes of victims of cyberbullying: the role of personal and contextual factors. J Sch Psychol. 2018;70:74–88.
45. Connell NM, et al. Badgrlz? Exploring sex differences in cyberbullying behaviors. Youth Violence and Juvenile Justice. 2014;12(3):209–28.
46. Cross D, et al.. Australian covert bullying prevalence study; 2009.
47. Li Q. Cyberbullying in schools: a research of gender differences. School Psychol Int. 2006;27(2):157–70.
48. Hemphill SA, Heerde JA. Adolescent predictors of young adult cyberbullying perpetration and victimization among Australian youth. J Adolescent Health. 2014;55(4):580–7.
49. Alhajji M, Bass S, Dai T. Cyberbullying, mental health, and violence in adolescents and associations with sex and race: data from the 2015 youth risk behavior survey. Glob Pediatr Health. 2019;6:2333794x19868887.
50. Navarro R, Yubero S, Larrañaga E. Cyberbullying across the globe: gender, family, and mental health. Springer; 2015.
51. Zych I, Ortega-Ruiz R, Del Rey R. Systematic review of theoretical studies on bullying and cyberbullying: facts, knowledge, prevention, and intervention. Aggression Violent Behav. 2015;23:1–21.
52. Hinduja S, Patchin JW. Personal information of adolescents on the Internet: a quantitative content analysis of MySpace. J Adolesc. 2008;31(1):125–46.
53. Slonje R, Smith PK. Cyberbullying: another main type of bullying? Scand J Psychol. 2008;49(2):147–54.
54. Ybarra ML, et al. Examining characteristics and associated distress related to Internet harassment: findings from the Second Youth Internet Safety Survey. Pediatrics. 2006;118(4):e1169–77.
55. McLoughlin LT, et al. Neurobiological underpinnings of cyberbullying: a pilot functional magnetic resonance imaging study. Hum Brain Mapp. 2020;41(6):1495–504.

6 Social Media and Cyberbullying

56. Chang FC, et al. Relationships among cyberbullying, school bullying, and mental health in Taiwanese adolescents. J Sch Health. 2013;83(6):454–62.
57. Kokkinos CM, Baltzidis E, Xynogala D. Prevalence and personality correlates of Facebook bullying among university undergraduates. Comput Human Behav. 2016;55:840–50.
58. Vitoroulis I, Vaillancourt T. Meta-analytic results of ethnic group differences in peer victimization. Aggress Behav. 2015;41(2):149–70.
59. Goebert D, et al. The impact of cyberbullying on substance use and mental health in a multiethnic sample. Matern Child Health J. 2011;15(8):1282–6.
60. Edwards L, Kontostathis AE, Fisher C. Cyberbullying, race/ethnicity and mental health outcomes: a review of the literature. Media Commun. 2016;4:71.
61. Wang J, Iannotti RJ, Nansel TR. School bullying among adolescents in the United States: physical, verbal, relational, and cyber. J Adolesc Health. 2009;45(4):368–75.
62. Cassidy W, Faucher C, Jackson M. Adversity in university: cyberbullying and its impacts on students, faculty and administrators. Int J Environ Res Public Health. 2017;14(8)
63. Alrajeh SM, et al. An investigation of the relationship between cyberbullying, cybervictimization and depression symptoms: a cross sectional study among university students in Qatar. PLoS One. 2021;16(12):e0260263.
64. Abreu RL, Kenny MC. Cyberbullying and LGBTQ Youth: a systematic literature review and recommendations for prevention and intervention. J Child Adolesc Trauma. 2018;11(1):81–97.
65. Albdour M, et al. The impact of cyberbullying on physical and psychological health of arab american adolescents. J Immigr Minor Health. 2019;21(4):706–15.
66. Viner RM, et al. Roles of cyberbullying, sleep, and physical activity in mediating the effects of social media use on mental health and wellbeing among young people in England: a secondary analysis of longitudinal data. Lancet Child Adolesc Health. 2019;3(10):685–96.
67. Kashy-Rosenbaum G, Aizenkot D. Exposure to cyberbullying in WhatsApp classmates‘ groups and classroom climate as predictors of students‘ sense of belonging: a multi-level analysis of elementary, middle and high schools. Children Youth Services Rev. 2020;108:104614.
68. Mitchell KJ, et al. What features make online harassment incidents upsetting to youth? J School Violence. 2016;15(3):279–301.
69. Kircaburun K, et al. Problematic online behaviors among adolescents and emerging adults: associations between cyberbullying perpetration, problematic social media use, and psychosocial factors. Int J Mental Health Addiction. 2019;17:891–908.
70. Giordano AL, Prosek EA, Watson JC. Understanding adolescent cyberbullies: exploring social media addiction and psychological factors. J Child Adolescent Counseling. 2021;7(1):42–55.
71. Saridakis G, et al. Individual information security, user behaviour and cyber victimisation: an empirical study of social networking users. Technol Forecasting Social Change. 2016;102:320–30.
72. Ho M, Quynh TT, Gu P, Chuanhua. Cyberbullying victimization and depression: self-esteem as a mediator and approach coping strategies as moderators. J Am College Health. 2021:1–8.
73. Liu C, Liu Z, Yuan G. The longitudinal influence of cyberbullying victimization on depression and posttraumatic stress symptoms: the mediation role of rumination. Arch Psychiatr Nurs. 2020;34(4):206–10.

Sexuality on the Internet: Identity Exploration, Cybersex and Sexting

7

Alice Caesar

Introduction

Adolescence is the stage when young people develop an interest in sex and start to explore their own sexual orientation and identity. In current times, the internet plays a central role in the adolescents' development of sexuality [1]. The percentage of teens who have smartphones has grown from 41% in 2012 to 89% in 2018 [2]. Sexting generally refers to the act of sending or receiving sexual texts or images. Since sexting is most often done via smartphones, this has likely contributed to rising rates of sexting among both teens and tweens [3].

Prevalence

The prevalence of sexting among adolescents varies widely across studies, from 7.6–60% for passive sexting (i.e., receiving pictures or texts) and 0.9–27.6% for active sexting (i.e., sending pictures or texts) [4]. Some of this variation is attributable to a lack of consensus among researchers as to the definition of sexting, with some defining it only as the sending of nude or partially nude photos and others more broadly as the sending, and receiving of both images or sexually suggestive texts [4]. Recent studies show much higher rates of sexting among teens today than ten years ago, likely fueled by the exponential growth of social media usage and smartphone ownership by adolescents over the past decade. Sexting is more common among older adolescence, with 30% of college freshman reporting having sent a nude photo during high school and 45% reporting receiving one [5].

A. Caesar (✉)
Department of Child and Adolescent Psychiatry, New York Presbyterian-Weill Cornell Medical College, New York, NY, USA
e-mail: alc9131@med.cornell.edu

© The Author(s), under exclusive license to Springer Nature Switzerland AG 2023
A. Spaniardi, J. M. Avari (eds.), *Teens, Screens, and Social Connection*,
https://doi.org/10.1007/978-3-031-24804-7_7

A meta-analysis conducted on the prevalence of sexting including data from 39 studies conducted during the period 2008–2016 found the mean prevalence for sending and receiving a sext was 14.8% and 27.4%, respectively. Prevalence increased with age of participant and year of study, with older adolescents more likely to send and receive sexts, and more recent studies showing higher rates than older studies. The prevalence of forwarding a sext without someone's consent was 12.5% and of having their sext forwarded without their consent was 8.4%. No significant difference was seen in the rates of sexting between males and females [3].

A 2013 survey of 1,208 Los Angeles High School Students who owned smartphones found that 17% of teens had both sent and received sexts, and 24% had only received sexts. Prevalence of sexting was again correlated with age, with older teens being more likely to sext. Sexting behavior was susceptible to peer influence, with teens who sexted being twice as likely to report knowing a peer who sexted, and teens who received a sext being thirteen times more likely to report knowing a peer who sexted [6].

Another study found similar rates of sexting in a sample of 622 private high school students. The rate of sending sexts was equal across genders (15.8% in males, 13.6% in females). The rate of receiving sexts was higher in males (40.5%) versus females (30.6%). The rates of forwarding sexts were 12.2% among males and 7.6% among females. Compared to data collected four years earlier, the rates of teens sending and receiving sexts were unchanged, but the rate of forwarding images had decreased by half (from 27.2% to 12.2% in males and 21.4% to 7.6% in females). In response to the previous study, the school had implemented several measures to combat sexting behavior. While the measures curbed the forwarding of sexts, it did not change sexting behavior. Adolescents continued to sext despite being educated regarding potential legal and psychosocial ramifications of sexting. Additionally, prevalence rates were stable across ages, suggesting that younger teens in this study were sexting as much as older teens [7].

Taken together, these three studies highlight that sexting is common among teens, and its presence should not be viewed as a sign of delinquency. Sexting has become a normative part of adolescent sexual development [4, 8]. Adolescence is a time of identity formation, in which teens start to separate from their family, and peer groups become more important. Sexual development is a critical part of identity formation in teens [9]. Youth are growing up in a digital age, and part of their sexual exploration is now occurring online.

The Experience of Sexting

Teens use the sending and receiving of sexual images, and exchange of explicit texts, as a way to flirt and form intimacy with partners [8]. Sixty-six percent of teens who sext report doing so because a date or significant other requested it, and 65% report sending it in hopes of attracting someone they like [5]. When the sending and receiving of sexual images happens in the context of a romantic relationship, it may not be linked to other high-risk behaviors (such as high-risk sexual behavior, alcohol use, marijuana use, or bullying) [10].

Sexting is highly associated with sexual intercourse [11, 12]. One study showed that adolescents who have sent or received sexual images were twice as likely to have had sex than those who haven't sent or received images (64.1% vs. 33%) [13]. Sexting is not utilized by teens as an alternative to sexual behavior, but rather as part of other sexual activities [6]. Sexting can sometimes proceed having sex (as a form of flirting) or happen concurrently (as a way to grow intimacy) [8].

When college students were asked to reflect back on their experience of sexting in high school, they described both good and bad experiences that "helped facilitate their growth and development and finding their sexual selves" [1]. Most adolescents who send nude or seminude photos describe it as a positive experience [5]. Positive outcomes from sexting include feeling beautiful, feeling attractive, exploring their sexuality, and getting closer to a romantic interest [14], as well as feeling more confident [2]. Rare negative outcomes include bullying, picture being forwarded without consent, and getting into legal trouble; all of these happened < 10% of the time. Although, school administrators, parents, and the media often focus on these risks, most teens don't experience these [14].

While most youth report positive experiences, some are at risk for negative outcomes from sexting. Sexting can trigger strong emotional reactions. Common negative outcomes from sexting include feeling anxious (49%), embarrassed (34%), or depressed (19%) [14]. The intensity of these emotions can worsen with time (34%) or remain unchanged (48%). Sexting can also make adolescents feel insecure about their body [1]. It's important to ask teens about their motivations for sexting, and what emotions sexting triggers both during the exchange and after [14]. Some adolescents may be more vulnerable to the potential negative effects of sexting, including girls, sexual minority youth, and those with mental health issues. Sexting can also be a marker for the presence of other impulsive behaviors, including risky sexual activity and drug use. As clinicians often work with teens who are vulnerable to potential negative outcomes from sexting, it is important that clinicians talk to patients about their online relationships.

Sexting in Younger Adolescents

Three studies have explored sexting behavior in younger adolescence [15]. Sexting in younger teens has been linked to increased sexual activity at a younger age, substance use, lack of parental supervision, and increased emotional problems.

Middle schoolers have significant exposure to sexting [11, 15]. A survey of Los Angeles middle schoolers found that 20% of students with text-capable cell phones had received a sext and 5% had sent a sext [11]. Another study showed young adolescents with emotional and behavioral problems had even higher rates of sexting behavior, with 17% reporting sending a sexual message and 5% reporting sending a sexual photo within the past six months. Both studies found that young adolescents who received or sent sexts were four to six times more likely to be sexually active than their peers [11, 15]. High rates of texting behavior in general were also independently linked to increased risk of being sexually active, suggesting one potential mediator for both texting and sexting in middle schoolers is decreased parental supervision [11]. Since increased risk of STDs and teen pregnancy is linked to younger age of first sexual activity, screening for sexting can identify at-risk youth [11].

Younger adolescents who sext are more likely to engage in other impulsive, risky behaviors such as consuming alcohol. Research from Europe found that younger girls who engaged in sexting were 10 times more likely to consume alcohol than their aged-matched peers who didn't sext. In comparison, the odds ratio for drinking alcohol in younger boys who sexted was 4.41, older girls was 2.89, and older boys was 1.66 [16].

Sexting at any age has been linked to increased emotional problems. However, this is more pronounced in younger adolescents. Younger girls and boys who sexted were almost three times more likely to struggle with emotional problems, while older girls and boys were two times more likely [16].

Developmentally, sexting is viewed differently based on age. Younger adolescents more often report doing it for "fun," to gain social status, or as part of a platonic relationship, while older youth report sexting to express romantic feelings or to maintain intimacy in a relationship [4, 16]. This may be why younger adolescents are at risk of greater harm from receiving sexts [17] and are more likely to be embarrassed or upset by sexting [4]. Youth who engage in sexting due to peer pressure or as a way to gain social status may be more vulnerable to feeling unfulfilled by sending and receiving sexual messages. They may also be more likely to engage in other risky behaviors based on peer pressure (such as sex, or substances). Engaging in sexting at a younger age should therefore be viewed as a red flag for the presence of other risky behaviors, emotional problems, or negative outcomes.

Gender Differences

Girls are more often negatively impacted by sexting than boys [4]. Girls are less likely to report feeling positively about themselves after sending a sext (14.5% vs. 30.7%) [7], and are more likely to report being harmed or embarrassed by receiving messages [17]. Girls are more likely to report nonconsensual sexting, and express feeling pressured to sext, with one study showing that about half of their sexting is driven by feeling pressured [5, 13]. Some studies have found that girls are more likely to send photos [5, 15, 18], and boys are more likely to receive photos [7], although this has not been replicated by all studies [6, 11]. Girls who feel pressured to send sexts are more likely to feel upset after the photo is sent [5]. Sending photos places girls at greater risk for those photos being forwarded without their consent, which can have broader legal and social consequences. There remains a society double-standard, in which girls are judged harshly for sending and receiving sexual images. Girls can be labeled "sluts" for sending images, and "prudes" for refusing to [19]. In contrast, boys are often immune from social criticism, and are socially rewarded for sending and receiving sexts [19, 20]. Acknowledging this double standard when discussing sexting with female patients is important. Conversations about sexting should include a broader dialogue about female sexuality and sensuality. These discussions should strive to empower young women to have ownership of their body, both physically and in print.

Sexual Minority Adolescents

Sexual minority adolescents (SMA) are more likely to engage in sexting than heterosexual youth [8, 18]. In the 2012 Youth Behavior Survey of Los Angeles middle school students, SMA were nine times more likely to have sent or received a sexually explicit photo than their gender-conforming peers [11]. Sexual minority youth are also more likely to feel coerced to send sexually explicit photos [21].

Geosocial networking applications (GNAs) (such as Tinder, Grindr, Scruff, and Jack'd) are social networking applications that use GPS to connect users. These apps provide a platform for the exchange of sexually explicit information and pictures, and facilitate users meeting in person through GPS: 53–70% of SMA males who are sexually active have used GNAs. For sexual minority youth, the internet can provide a safe space for exploration of gender and identity. However, it also leaves them vulnerable to be taken advantage of by older adults. Sexual minority youth who use GNAs are at risk for being stalked, engaging in unprotected sex, and experiencing sexual violence [22]. Clinicians who work with SMA have a unique opportunity to counsel adolescents about these risks. It is important to ask teens about their online partner seeking. Exploring and validating their motivation for seeking out online relationships is important, while also counseling them on potential risks and how to stay safe online. Clinicians should also direct them to more age-appropriate safe spaces to explore their sexuality and identity. The Trevor Project's TrevorSpace is one option, which offers a moderated space for SMA (https://www.trevorspace.org/) [22].

Mental Health Concerns

Adolescents with psychological and emotional problems report two to three fold higher rates of engaging in sexting [16], and are more vulnerable to potential emotional repercussions. Engaging in sexting has been linked to low self-esteem [15, 18]. Two studies have found that sexting is more common in girls who endorse depressive symptoms [18, 23]. Youth with psychological difficulties are more likely to report being harmed from receiving sexual images [17].

Teens who experience nonconsensual sexting are at even higher risk for psychological and emotional problems. Nonconsensual sexting occurs when one participant feels pressured, or coerced, to send a nude or seminude photo, or when a photo is forwarded without consent. The 2015 Pennsylvania Youth Risk Behavior Survey found that consensual sexting was related to multiple mental health variables including serious depressive symptoms (39.8% vs. 27.8%), attempting suicide (14.6% vs. 6.7%), and engaging in self-harm behavior in past year (27% vs. 19.3%).

When sexting was nonconsensual, the relationship was even more concerning, with higher rates of serious depressive symptoms (43%), attempting suicide (27.5%), and self-harm behavior (52.1%) [13].

Adolescents with psychological and emotional problems may feel more pressure to share private photos as a way to gain intimacy, or social approval, and may also be more sensitive to potential rejection if the sharing doesn't fulfill their expectations. This may be most pronounced in younger girls [16].

Sexting and the Link to Risky Behavior

The presence of sexting can be a marker for other impulsive behaviors, and should prompt clinicians to screen for additional high-risk activities. Sexting may highlight underlying issues in impulse control [6–8], and has been associated with sensation seeking, alcohol use, and substance use [8, 13, 16, 18, 23]. Receiving sexually explicit images has been linked to increased risk-taking behavior both online and offline [17].

Sexting is highly correlated with engaging in other sexual activities. Middle school teens who sext are five times more likely to be having vaginal sex than their peers [15]. Active sexting (i.e., sending a nude photo) may be a predictor for becoming sexually active in the next year [8]. Adolescents who share sexual photos are more likely to be having all forms of sex (anal, oral, and vaginal) [18]. Sexting has been linked to engaging in risky sexual behaviors, such as having many sexual partners within the past year or concurrent partners [18], as well as having unprotected sex [6]. Adolescents who sext may also be at increased risk for sexual victimization and intimate partner violence [24]. Consensual and nonconsensual sexting is related to a two-fold and four-fold increased risk of experiencing sexual dating violence, respectively (13.9% if sexting is consensual vs. 25.4% if sexting is nonconsensual vs. 6.1% overall risk for all teens in sample) [13]. Disclosure of sexting by youth should therefore be seen as an opportunity for clinicians to counsel patients on safe sex practices, contraception, STDs, and sexual trauma.

Given the increasing prevalence of sexting, though, it is clear that not all teens who sext are engaging in additional impulsive behaviors. More research is needed to clarify the association between sexting and other high-risk behaviors. Sexting has been highly correlated with becoming sexually active in the next year; however, it did not show a relationship with engaging in risky sexual behavior, having multiple sexual partners, or consuming alcohol or marijuana prior to sex [8]. Similarly, sexting within a romantic relationship is not correlated with other high-risk behaviors (such as alcohol use, marijuana use, high-risk sexual behavior, or bullying) [10]. Although, sexting can be correlated with risky behaviors, it is important for clinicians to appreciate that more often sexting is a normative part of adolescent sexual activity [8]. When sexting occurs within a romantic relationship as a way to grow intimacy and explore their sexuality, it likely is not a marker for other high-risk or deviant behaviors.

Legal Risks

The potential legal implications of sexting vary greatly state to state. Given the growing prevalence of this behavior, many states have moved to decriminalize the exchange of consensual teen to teen sharing of sexually explicit images. In almost half of the United States, though, teens who engage in sexting can still be prosecuted, convicted, and sentenced to up to 20 years in prison and receive a lifetime sexual offender status for production and possession of child pornography. Although prosecution of adolescents is rare, it is important to educate teens on the risk of legal consequences for consensual, nonconsensual, and coerced sexting [25].

Conclusion and Tips for Clinicians

Adolescence is a time of identity formation and sexual exploration. With the growth of technology and smartphones, the internet is playing a greater role in this development. Sexting has become a normative part of teen's exploration of their sexual identity and sensuality, and for many, it is a positive experience. Clinicians who work with teenagers have the unique opportunity of providing a safe, nonjudgmental space for adolescents to share their experiences.

It is helpful for clinicians to talk to adolescents about their online activities. Exploring with them how they feel about themselves before, during, and after sexting is important. This can facilitate a broader discussion about their self-esteem and body image. Openly discussing what they hope to gain from sexting, whether it's greater intimacy in their relationship, improved social standing with friends, or alleviation of peer pressure, is significant. Asking about an adolescent's motivation for sexting can help teens reflect on their behavior, and potentially spur change.

When appropriate, clinicians can further screen adolescents at risk of negative fallout from sexting. Potentially vulnerable adolescents include younger teens, girls, sexual minority youth, and those with psychological or emotional problems. For these patients, it is important to ask about their online relationships; if they are engaging in sexting, clinicians can inquire as to whether it has been a positive or negative experience.

Since sexting is correlated with having sex, clinicians should also be counseling patients on safe sex, and risk for STDs. It is important to talk to teens about the physical danger of meeting people in-person who they've been talking to online, and risks of intimate partner violence. As sexting can be associated with other high-risk behavior, clinicians should screen and counsel adolescents on alcohol and substance use.

Conversations about sexting should occur in the setting of a larger dialogue about sex, intimacy, sexuality, and sensuality. The ultimate goal is not to judge or shame, but rather to empower them to have ownership of their body both physically, as well as in print and in word.

Key Points
- Youth are growing up in a digital age and part of their sexual exploration is now occurring online.
- Some adolescents may be more vulnerable to the potential negative effects of sexting, including girls, sexual minority youth, and those with mental health issues.
- The presence of sexting can be a marker for other impulsive behaviors, and should prompt clinicians to screen for additional high-risk activities.
- Sexting carries with it potential legal implications.

Multiple Choice Questions
1. What factor has consistently been found to increase the prevalence of sexting?
   A. Age
   B. Gender
   C. Popularity
   D. Socioeconomic status
   Correct Answer: A
2. Sexting has been highly correlated with:
   A. Poor academic performance
   B. Engaging in risky sexual behavior
   C. Having multiple sexual partners
   D. Becoming sexually active in the next year
   Correct Answer: D
3. The presence of sexting can be a marker for:
   A. Delinquency
   B. Sexual Abuse
   C. Impulsive Behaviors
   D. Major Depressive Disorder
   Correct Answer: C

References

1. Murphy DM, Spencer B. Teens' experiences with sexting: a grounded theory study. J Pediatr Health Care. 2021;35(4):387–400. https://doi.org/10.1016/j.pedhc.2020.11.010.
2. Anderson M, Jiang J. Teens, social media & technology 2018. Pew Research Center; 2018.
3. Madigan S, Ly A, Rash CL, Van Ouytsel J, Temple JR. Prevalence of multiple forms of sexting behavior among youth: a systematic review and meta-analysis. JAMA Pediatr. 2018;172(4):327–35. https://doi.org/10.1001/jamapediatrics.2017.5314.
4. Barrense-Dias Y, Berchtold A, Suris JC, Akre C. Sexting and the definition issue. J Adolesc Health. 2017;61(5):544–54. https://doi.org/10.1016/j.jadohealth.2017.05.009.
5. Englander E. Low risk associated with most teenage sexting: a study of 617 18-year-olds. Massachusetts Aggression Reduction Center; 2012, http://webhost.bridgew.edu/marc/SEXTING%20AND%20COERCION%20report.pdf.
6. Rice E, Craddock J, Hemler M, Rusow J, Plant A, Montoya J, Kordic T. Associations between sexting behaviors and sexual behaviors among mobile phone-owning teens in Los Angeles. Child Dev. 2018;89(1):110–7. https://doi.org/10.1111/cdev.12837.

7. Strassberg DS, Cann D, Velarde V. Sexting by high school students. Arch Sex Behav. 2017;46(6):1667–72. https://doi.org/10.1007/s10508-016-0926-9.
8. Temple JR, Choi H. Longitudinal association between teen sexting and sexual behavior. Pediatrics. 2014;134(5):e1287–92. https://doi.org/10.1542/peds.2014-1974.
9. Erikson EH. Childhood and society. 2nd ed. New York: Norton; 1963.
10. Van Ouytsel J, Walrave M, Lu Y, Temple JR, Ponnet K. The associations between substance use, sexual behavior, deviant behaviors and adolescents' engagement in sexting: does relationship context matter? J Youth Adolesc. 2018;47(11):2353–70. https://doi.org/10.1007/s10964-018-0903-9.
11. Rice E, Gibbs J, Winetrobe H, Rhoades H, Plant A, Montoya J, Kordic T. Sexting and sexual behavior among middle school students. Pediatrics. 2014;134(1):e21–8. https://doi.org/10.1542/peds.2013-2991.
12. Temple JR, Paul JA, van den Berg P, Le VD, McElhany A, Temple BW. Teen sexting and its association with sexual behaviors. Arch Pediatr Adolesc Med. 2012;166(9):828–33. https://doi.org/10.1001/archpediatrics.2012.835.
13. Frankel AS, Bass SB, Patterson F, Dai T, Brown D. Sexting, risk behavior, and mental health in adolescents: an examination of 2015 Pennsylvania Youth Risk Behavior Survey Data. J Sch Health. 2018;88(3):190–9. https://doi.org/10.1111/josh.12596.
14. Englander E. Sexting before and during the pandemic, online; 2021.
15. Houck CD, Barker D, Rizzo C, Hancock E, Norton A, Brown LK. Sexting and sexual behavior in at-risk adolescents. Pediatrics. 2014;133(2):e276–82. https://doi.org/10.1542/peds.2013-1157.
16. Ševčíková A. Girls' and boys' experience with teen sexting in early and late adolescence. J Adolesc. 2016;51:156–62. https://doi.org/10.1016/j.adolescence.2016.06.007.
17. Livingstone S, Görzig A. When adolescents receive sexual messages on the internet: explaining experiences of risk and harm. Comput Human Behav. 2014;33:8–15. https://doi.org/10.1016/j.chb.2013.12.021.
18. Ybarra ML, Mitchell KJ. "Sexting" and its relation to sexual activity and sexual risk behavior in a national survey of adolescents. J Adolesc Health. 2014;55(6):757–64. https://doi.org/10.1016/j.jadohealth.2014.07.012.
19. Lippman JR, Campbell SW. Damned if you do, damned if you don't…if you're a girl: relational and normative contexts of adolescent sexting in the United States. J Children Media. 2014;8:371–86.
20. Ringrose J, Regehr K, Whitehead S. Teen girls' experiences negotiating the ubiquitous dick pic: sexual double standards and the normalization of image based sexual harassment. Sex Roles. 2021;1–19. https://doi.org/10.1007/s11199-021-01236-3.
21. Van Ouytsel J, Walrave M, Ponnet K. An exploratory study of sexting behaviors among heterosexual and sexual minority early adolescents. J Adolesc Health. 2019;65(5):621–6. https://doi.org/10.1016/j.jadohealth.2019.06.003.
22. Suto DJ, Macapagal K, Turban JL. Geosocial networking application use among sexual minority adolescents. J Am Acad Child Adolesc Psychiatry. 2021;60(4):429–31. https://doi.org/10.1016/j.jaac.2020.11.018.
23. Van Ouytsel J, Van Gool E, Ponnet K, Walrave M. Brief report: the association between adolescents' characteristics and engagement in sexting. J Adolesc. 2014;37(8):1387–91. https://doi.org/10.1016/j.adolescence.2014.10.004.
24. Titchen KE, Maslyanskaya S, Silver EJ, Coupey SM. Sexting and young adolescents: associations with sexual abuse and intimate partner violence. J Pediatr Adolesc Gynecol. 2019;32(5):481–6. https://doi.org/10.1016/j.jpag.2019.07.004.
25. Strasburger VC, Zimmerman H, Temple JR, Madigan S. Teenagers, sexting, and the law. Pediatrics. 2019;143(5). https://doi.org/10.1542/peds.2018-3183.

Internet Gaming Disorder and Addictive Behaviors Online

8

Alex El Sehamy and Pantea Farahmand

Introduction

Though not an official diagnosis in the Diagnostic and Statistical Manual of Mental Disorders (DSM), Internet Gaming Disorder (IGD) has been included in the DSM-5 as a "Condition for Further Study." This classification suggests that the diagnosis is not yet intended for clinical use, but that research on the topic is encouraged. Epidemiological research has yielded a variety of statistics on the prevalence of IGD, which is likely attributable to various definitions of the disorder over the years, regional differences, and different methods of assessment. A large meta-analysis yielded a 1.96% to 3.05% global prevalence among all age groups [1] and another meta-analysis of sixteen studies yielded a 4.6% prevalence rate among adolescents with 6.8% prevalence for males and 1.3% prevalence for females [2]. Not only is problematic internet gaming highly prevalent in our society, but it comes with significant biopsychosocial impacts as well. Children aged 8–10 spend eight hours per day using various electronic media recreationally and adolescents spend more than eleven hours per day doing the same, which is more time than they spend in school or with friends [3]. A recent meta-analysis revealed that problematic gaming was significantly associated with 20.8 min less sleep per night on average, a 1.5-fold increased risk of daytime sleepiness, and more than double the risk of poorer sleep quality and sleep problems [4]. Due to statistics such as these, the concept of IGD gained significant attention from experts in East Asian countries who began supporting education, research, and treatment [5]. China had even implemented nationwide restrictions in 2019 on internet gaming for adolescents due to the growing public health threat, which were later tightened even further in 2021 [6]. Though a

---

A. El Sehamy (✉) · P. Farahmand
Department of Child and Adolescent Psychiatry, NYU Child Study Center, NYU Grossman School of Medicine, New York, NY, USA
e-mail: Alexander.Elsehamy@nyulangone.org; pantea.farahmand@nyulangone.org

© The Author(s), under exclusive license to Springer Nature Switzerland AG 2023
A. Spaniardi, J. M. Avari (eds.), *Teens, Screens, and Social Connection*,
https://doi.org/10.1007/978-3-031-24804-7_8

relatively new phenomenon in the context of human history, "internet addiction" has been a concern of mental health professionals since the inception of the World Wide Web.

The earliest known research on this topic dates back to 1996 when Kimberly Young sought to verify a set of criteria to distinguish "addictive" internet usage from "normal" internet usage [7]. She used a brief eight-item Diagnostic Questionnaire (DQ) which modified criteria for pathological gambling to use as a screening instrument for addictive internet use in adults. A cut-off score of five items was used, consistent with the threshold for pathological gambling.

1. *Do you feel preoccupied with the Internet (think about previous on-line activity or anticipate next on-line session)?*
2. *Do you feel the need to use the Internet with increasing amounts of time in order to achieve satisfaction?*
3. *Have you repeatedly made unsuccessful efforts to control, cut back, or stop Internet use?*
4. *Do you feel restless, moody, depressed, or irritable when attempting to cut down or stop Internet use?*
5. *Do you stay on-line longer than originally intended?*
6. *Have you jeopardized or risked the loss of significant relationship, job, educational or career opportunity because of the Internet?*
7. *Have you lied to family members, therapist, or others to conceal the extent of involvement with the Internet?*
8. *Do you use the Internet as a way of escaping from problems or of relieving a dysphoric mood (e.g., feelings of helplessness, guilt, anxiety, depression)?*

As the internet and consumer computing technology was still in very early stages at this time, Young's initial results would be an important reference point for future research in the field. She notably observed that a significant majority of those meeting criteria (or "dependents") were female (239 females versus 157 males) and that 42% of the entire sample of dependents was unemployed (homemakers, disabled, retired, or students). Additionally, 63% of dependents rated their most utilized internet applications were chat rooms and multiuser dungeons (text-based role-playing games) as opposed to news reading, e-mailing, and web surfing. Though this study has many limitations including selection bias and lack of generalizability, it was a landmark study that suggests both direct peer-to-peer communication and gaming have long been very important and potentially problematic features of internet usage.

Symptomatology and Controversy

Let's take a closer look at the proposed criteria for IGD in the DSM-5:

Persistent and recurrent use of the internet to engage in games, often with other players, leading to clinically significant impairment or distress as indicated by five (or more) of the following in a 12-month period:

1. *Preoccupation with Internet games. (The individual thinks about previous gaming activity or anticipates playing the next game; Internet gaming becomes the dominant activity in daily life). Note: This disorder is distinct from Internet gaming, which is included under gambling disorder.*
2. *Withdrawal symptoms when Internet gaming is taken away. (These symptoms are typically described as irritability, anxiety, or sadness, but there are no physical signs of pharmacological withdrawal.)*
3. *Tolerance: the need to spend increasing amounts of time engaged in Internet games.*
4. *Unsuccessful attempts to control the participation in Internet games.*
5. *Loss of interests in previous hobbies and entertainment as a result of, and with the exception of, Internet games.*
6. *Continued excessive use of Internet games despite knowledge of psychosocial problems.*
7. *Has deceived family members, therapists, or others regarding the amount of Internet gaming.*
8. *Use of Internet games to escape or relieve a negative mood (e.g., feelings of helplessness, guilt, anxiety).*
9. *Has jeopardized or lost a significant relationship, job, or education or career opportunity because of participation in Internet games.*

As seen in Table 8.1, the criteria for IGD overlap somewhat with criteria for a substance-use disorder and largely with the criteria for gambling disorder (an X indicates the disorder has a similar criterion for diagnosis). The gambling disorder criteria that replace numbers 5 and 6 for IGD are more specific to gambling behavior (chasing losses and relying on other financially) and overall only four or more of the total criteria are required for diagnosis. For all substance-use disorders only two criterion are required for diagnosis. As we examine the admission of addictive behaviors into the DSM, we observe a tendency to raise the threshold for diagnosis. Controversy over pathologizing normal human behavior is widespread in the literature on IGD. In a 2017 editorial [8], Markey and Ferguson expound upon a

Table 8.1 *Diagnostic and Statistical Manual of Mental Disorders,* revision 5, Internet gaming disorder criteria and their relation to substance use and gambling disorder criteria

Internet gaming disorder criteria	Substance-use disorder criteria	Gambling disorder criteria
Preoccupation with playing	–	X
Withdrawal symptoms when not playing	X	X
Tolerance	X	X
Unsuccessful attempts to reduce or stop playing	X	X
Gives up other activities to play	X	–
Continues playing despite problems caused by it	X	–
Deceives or covers up playing	–	X
Plays to escape adverse moods	–	X
Risks or loses relationships or career opportunities because of excessive playing	–	X

large-scale 2017 survey study by Przybylski et al [9] and present numerous points in support of re-examining the current proposed DSM-5 criteria for IGD as outlined below:

1. *The prevalence of Internet gaming disorder was lower among people who played a video game in the last year than the prevalence of gambling disorder among people who had engaged in any form of gambling in the past year.*
2. *Those meeting the criteria for diagnosis of Internet gaming disorder did not display any differences in terms of behavioral or clinical effects.*
3. *The biggest difference found was that those who were diagnosed as having the disorder simply played more video games than other individuals.*

The results from Przybylski et al and the subsequent controversy raise an important point about the phenomenon of video gaming and how we define it as a disordered or problematic behavior. The truth of the matter is that as of 2013, there were at least 18 different ways in which researchers have operationalized Internet gaming disorder [10]. Markey and Ferguson were also concerned with the homogeneity of clinical weight given to each diagnostic criterion for IGD, as is standard practice with all diagnoses in the DSM. They argue that a case in which an individual who loses a job or personal relationship due to being unable to stop playing video games is fundamentally different from a case in which someone plays video games to escape negative moods and loses interest in other, less effective hobbies. The higher threshold for diagnosis when compared to gambling disorder or substance-use disorders surely addresses some concerns for overdiagnosis and stigmatization. However, in caring for the child and adolescent population, it would behoove us to take the findings in this very new area of research with a grain of salt.

Participants in Przybylski's study were at youngest 18 years of age. Due to the myriad biopsychosocial variables present in the life of a child or adolescent and the critical nature of these formative years of life, the relative consequences of IGD for a child (school truancy, strained parental/social relationships) could potentially carry a higher individual and societal disease burden. If we consider how these behavioral consequences of IGD might have longitudinal effects on a child's development, we can begin to understand the need for specific research in the pediatric population. That being said, discovering general ways to predict severity or prognosis based on symptomatology can be an important tool for clinical management.

Using a tree-based model that operationalized IGD criteria as continuous rather than binary variables, researchers were able to define subgroups of disordered gamers (mean age = 20 years, SD = 4.3 years) based on different characteristics [11]. Their analysis revealed that "withdrawal," "loss of control," "negative consequences," and "preoccupation" were key predictors of an IGD diagnosis. They were able to create subgroups and attribute them to clusters of these characteristics as follows: "Impaired Self-Control" (withdrawal and loss of control), "Harmful" (withdrawal, loss of control, and negative consequences), "Preoccupied" (withdrawal and preoccupation). Falling within each subgroup increased likelihood of an IGD diagnosis by 77.77%, 26.66%, and 7.14% respectively. Withdrawal being a

8 Internet Gaming Disorder and Addictive Behaviors Online

core feature of these subgroups is a finding congruent with seminal work by Charlton and Danforth [12, 13] and their claims of "core" and "peripheral" criteria in the diagnosis of IGD have been corroborated by several follow-up studies [14–17]. Yet in 2018, the World Health Organization (WHO) released the 11th International Classification of Diseases (ICD-11), which included a Gaming Disorder (GD) diagnosis with criteria completely devoid of the phenomenon of withdrawal [18]. According to the ICD-11, GD can pertain to online or offline gaming and is diagnosed by meeting the following criteria:

1. *Impaired control over gaming (e.g., onset, frequency, intensity, duration, termination, context).*
2. *Increasing priority given to gaming to the extent that gaming takes precedence over other life interests and daily activities.*
3. *Continuation or escalation of gaming despite the occurrence of negative consequences.*
4. *The behavior pattern is of sufficient severity to result in significant impairment in personal, family, social, educational, occupational, or other important areas of functioning.*

Certainly, less criteria can lead to overdiagnosis and this disparity between the ICD and DSM can be problematic for both research protocols and clinical management. Mental health professionals should remain judicious about diagnosis to avoid mismanagement and stigmatization of video gaming in society as there can actually be many advantages to video gaming (see "Recommendations" section).

Screening

Two years after the introduction of IGD into the DSM-5 in 2013, Korean researchers launched the Internet user Cohort for Unbiased Recognition of gaming disorder in Early Adolescence (iCURE) study with the aim to clarify the natural and clinical courses of IGD in adolescents and to evaluate risk and protective factors [19]. Using this carefully selected sample, the same researchers sought to understand how a self-assessment tool would fare against their multiple rounds of clinical diagnostic interviews. Unsurprisingly, the false-negative rate was 44% and the false-positive rate was 9.6%, resulting in a 56.6% sensitivity and 90.4% specificity of the self-assessment questionnaire [20]. Children were found to be minimizing their behavior much like a substance user would due to the social stigma surrounding their behavior.

The screening instruments that have been developed for IGD have shown variable efficacy. A systematic review of 320 studies with both adult and adolescent participants found greater evidential support for five out of thirty-two total tools [21]:

Assessment of Internet and Computer Addiction Scale-Gaming (AICA-Sgaming)
Game Addiction Scale-7 (GAS-7)
Internet Gaming Disorder Test-10 items (IGDT-10)

Internet Gaming Disorder Scale-9 Short Form (IGDS9-SF)
Internet Gaming Disorder Scale-9 items (Lemmens IGD-9)

According to the review, the GAS-7 was most frequently rated positively due to its large evidence base, which provides good criterion validity as well as internal and test-retest reliability. However, the GAS-7 has not been used in any clinical samples, whereas the AICA-Sgaming has and may hold some utility as an outcome measure in treatment. Additionally the GAS-7 has incomplete coverage for DSM-5 and ICD-11 criteria, which may not be essential for screening purposes but is important when considering its use as a diagnostic tool. The IGDS9-SF and IGDT-10 on the other hand do provide total coverage of the DSM-5 and ICD-11 criteria.

The discrepancy in DSM-5 and ICD-11 criteria along with the increasing need to identify at-risk adolescents has resulted in the development of even shorter screening tools. The Three-item Gaming disorder Test-Online-Centered, or TIGTOC, is composed of three items on a four-point Likert scale. The same researchers who created the aforementioned iCURE study analyzed their data to test the validity of this new ultra-brief screening tool and found a sensitivity of 72%, a specificity of 90%, and positive associations with time spent online gaming, depressive symptoms, attention-deficit/hyperactivity disorder symptoms, and addictive Internet use [22]. The TIGTOC may prove useful for emergency psychiatric and primary care settings where time is of the essence and management is often largely based on making appropriate referrals.

Risk and Protective Factors

A recent study published in the Journal of Child Psychology and Psychiatry used a novel statistical method called Random Intercept Cross-lagged Panel Modeling to examine the concurrent and prospective links between prevalence of IGD and prevalence of common psychiatric disorders in adolescents. They found only one link in their analysis: increased IGD symptoms at ages 10 and 12 predicted decreased symptoms of anxiety two years later. They otherwise concluded that observed co-occurrence between IGD symptoms and mental health problems can be mainly attributed to common underlying factors between adolescents [23]. In contrast, the same researchers who created the iCURE research protocol found that playing online games for over 240 min per day in addition to prevalence of ADHD symptoms were predictors of persistence of high-risk status in adolescents [24].

While causation is unclear, the literature emphasizes the importance of addressing this specific population with research and treatment protocols. A unique cohort study performed across several European countries found that adolescents who screened positive for problematic internet gaming showed significantly more signs of depression, conduct disorder, hyperactivity, issues with peers, perceived stress, and self-injurious behavior compared with adolescents who screened positive for problematic internet usage unrelated to gaming [25]. Playing single-player video games has also been found to mediate IGD severity [24]. Therefore, the population of adolescents participating specifically in online multiplayer gaming appears to be particularly at risk.

In examining the moderating effect of environmental factors on the development and prevalence of IGD in children specifically, researchers have discovered that affiliation with deviant peers seems to bolster the already existing correlation between sensation-seeking behavior and problematic internet usage, yet parental knowledge of their children's activities moderates and weakens these associations (Fig. 8.1) [26]. Thus, it should come as no surprise that single parent families are associated with increase in screen time of adolescents, as are parents who are characterized as "ignorant, oppressive, or hostile" [27]. Similarly, poor relationships with peers have also been shown to increase the risk of IGD in adolescents [28] and limited social and emotion regulation skills at age 8 have been shown to predict more IGD symptoms at age 10 [29].

These disrupted family relationships are also linked to disconnectivity within the reward circuit on resting state MRI [30]. Disconnectivity was found specifically between the right-middle frontal gyrus and the caudate and between the left cingulate and the caudate nucleus, which is consistent with previous research on children with attention-deficit hyperactivity disorder (ADHD), implying that children with IGD and those with ADHD may share some common pathophysiology [31]. Much of the research on psychiatric comorbidity with IGD focuses on ADHD due to the biopsychosocial correlates discussed here and treatment has proven effective (see section on Treatment and Prevention). Underlying psychiatric disorders can contribute to maladaptive or addictive behaviors and as such should always be a focus of treatment if present.

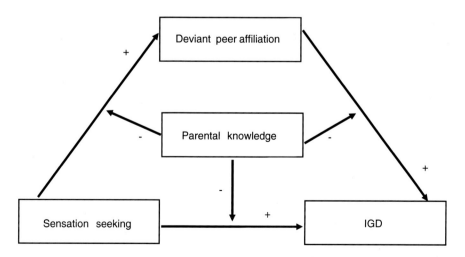

Fig. 8.1 Mediating effect of parental knowledge on sensation seeking, deviant peer affiliation, and IGD

Treatment and Prevention

As mentioned throughout this chapter, problematic internet use has been correlated with underlying mental health problems and treatments available today for IGD and other internet addictions emphasize providing treatment for underlying co-morbidities. According to a recent systematic review [32], several studies to date have found significant and sustained benefit from both psychological and pharmacological treatments. According to the review, psychotropic medications studied for treatment of internet addiction are those targeting depression, anxiety or ADHD while cognitive behavioral therapies (group and individual) are the cornerstone of evidence-based psychological treatments. Supportive group therapy, virtual reality group therapy, family therapy, eclectic therapy, and motivational therapy, among others may hold promise but have less evidence supporting their use [32]. More high-quality studies are needed to fully appreciate the relationship between IGD and co-occurring mental illness, in addition to further solidifying the evidence base of available treatments. However, in this section, we will discuss the current modalities used for treatment and prevention.

Antidepressant medications studied for treatment of IGD include bupropion and escitalopram. A pre-posttest designed study of bupropion SR in young adults found reduced craving for internet gaming, decreased play time, and decreased cue-induced brain activity in the dorsolateral prefrontal cortex after 6 weeks of treatment [33]. Another pre-posttest study of bupropion found reduced depressive symptoms, improved attention, decreased impulsivity, and reduced addictive measures on the Young Internet Addiction Scale (YIAS-K) after 12 weeks of treatment [34]. One study compared escitalopram and bupropion head-to-head after 12 weeks of treatment for excessive internet gaming and found clinical improvements in IGD symptoms but no significant differences between the two drugs [35]. Two randomized controlled trials also found positive results. An 8-week study showed statistically significant reduction in gaming and IGD symptoms in those treated with bupropion versus placebo [36]. A 6-week study found statistically significant reductions in IGD symptoms versus the control group [37]. Reductions were greater in the bupropion group than the escitalopram group.

Methylphenidate and atomoxetine are among the most studied ADHD-specific treatments in IGD research. An 8-week trial of methylphenidate in children diagnosed with ADHD found internet usage time and YIAS-K scores to be significantly reduced [38]. Additionally, a 12-week head to head study methylphenidate versus atomoxetine found reduced IGD symptoms, but no significant differences between the medications [39].

Most of the nonpharmacological IGD treatments studied are based on principles of cognitive behavioral therapy (CBT). Treatments include mindfulness strategies [40], CBT with parent psychoeducation, gaming-specific CBT, craving-focused CBT, and standard CBT. Head-to-head studies comparing the different types of CBT have not been extensively explored. Two comparison studies used non-randomized controlled designs. In one comparison study of individual CBT versus CBT with parent psychoeducation, both were found to decrease IGD symptoms.

Adding the parent psychoeducation, however, did not improve outcomes [41]. Another study comparing specialized CBT for IGD with standard CBT also found decreased IGD symptoms in both groups that were maintained at 3-month follow up. In this case though, the specialized CBT for IGD had statistically significantly improved outcomes compared to the standard CBT [42]. Three studies of CBT interventions were randomized controlled trials. These studies compared CBT group therapy with basic counseling for adolescents, mindfulness-oriented group therapy with supportive group therapy, and CBT group therapy with virtual reality group [43–45]. Though there were no statistically significant differences between these treatments, mindfulness-oriented group therapy was found to be superior to supportive group therapy. These studies found improved outcomes on posttreatment follow-up. One multicenter randomized clinical trial conducted with adult male participants found a short-term manualized CBT program to yield statistically greater remission rates versus the control group [36].

Combination behavioral and pharmacological intervention has been studied, but more research is needed to prove effectiveness. One randomized controlled study of adolescents found that the addition of CBT improved the effects of bupropion compared with bupropion alone in overall gaming time and IGD symptoms at 4 weeks post treatment [46].

Other treatment approaches that have been found to have benefits in decreasing gaming time and IGD symptoms include family therapy, transcranial direct current stimulation, and eclectic treatment that includes CBT, motivational interviewing, and solution-focused therapy. Reduced gaming time was also reported with a 9-day self-discovery camp program [47, 48]. Most of these studies are pre-post designs without randomization or control comparisons. One controlled comparison study compared a 7-day residential camp, 8 sessions of parent management, residential camp with parent management, and psychoeducation alone (control group). The three non-control groups were all superior to the control group and had sustained improvements on follow up [49].

Recommendations for Parents

Historically, fairy tales were used to help children process frightening content like abandonment, murder, and cannibalism in order to develop potentially life-saving skills. Victorian-era parents acknowledged that children would inevitably confront difficult situations and recognized that they should learn to master them. In today's world, the trend seems to be for "good" parents to limit their children's exposure to "negative" emotions and protect them from sadness or fear rather than celebrate their ability to cope with and overcome these emotions and situations. Video games can provide children with a safe space to explore these difficult emotions similarly to reading a fairy tale or playing a pretend game. As compared with real life or a movie, a video game allows players more control over emotions; players can choose situations to elicit, avoid, or indulge in particular feelings [50]. As such, video games may actually be less 'shocking' or 'traumatizing' than film or television programs as the child maintains some element of control. Qualitative research shows that video gaming can also serve as a bonding experience for children to share their identity with others or as a space to safely indulge in behaviors that one's family or community deems shameful or wrong [51]. An adolescent may be drawn to violent games to, for example, act out an extreme version of powerful masculinity safe from the judgment of parents or society [52] or to explore feminine behaviors and identities safely.

Researchers have outlined practical methods that parents can use in the home to identify and prevent problematic online video gaming. During a 2021 presentation at the American Academy of Child and Adolescent Psychiatry's Annual Meeting, Weigle and Englander discussed the trials and tribulations of parenting a child on the autism spectrum who may be showing signs of having internet gaming disorder as well. They recommend always transitioning them from video gaming to another very highly pleasurable activity to prevent aggression or agitation [53]. A qualitative study on children's motivations for video gaming also yielded important information for parents [51]. Increasing one's video game literacy can help a parent identify games, which may be more addictive (see Conclusion) or contain harmful themes (racial stereotypes, unrealistic body proportions, etc.). Restricting video game usage to common areas of the home such as the living room or den can also help to ensure that parents are aware of how long and how frequent children are gaming. Lastly, playing video games with children is a way to reduce the need for children to use video gaming as an escape from their home life. As much as 50% of children reported never having played video games with a parent. With the advent of more family friendly systems with more intuitive controls, a larger demographic can now enjoy gaming. Asking children to give instructions on how to play a game they are passionate about implies a respect for a child's interests and skills in a society that often dismisses video gaming as a pointless activity.

Associated Syndromes and Behaviors

Social Media

Social media use is a highly polarizing issue in our society with many opining that ubiquitous use of social media by adolescents has led to increasing rates of depression, anxiety, and eating disorders. A systematic review performed in 2020 classified four domains of social media use: time spent, activity, investment, and addiction, and found that all domains correlated with depression, anxiety, and psychological distress [54]. Eating disorder symptoms increase with greater social media use, particularly picture sharing-based apps, and some websites even advocate for eating disorders as a lifestyle rather than a disorder [55]. Pro-recovery content is often rare. Shockingly, children have been found to have significant disordered eating cognitions and behaviors as early as 7th grade [56]. Given that social media usage is covered in different contexts throughout the rest of this book, this section will focus solely on problematic or addictive social media use.

With the advent of the internet and social media, it is imperative to understand that there has been a cultural shift in the way children and adolescents view social activity. Additionally, parent's perceptions of their children and their social behaviors may be biased by their degree of anxiety or the safety of their local neighborhood, with some probably preferring children to be online rather than out in the world. In navigating this complicated new social paradigm and the possibility of addiction, we must consider the same symptoms emphasized for other types of addictive behavior (preoccupation, mood modification, tolerance, withdrawal, relapse, loss of control, and social/occupational functioning). However, upon a survey of the literature, it appears that research is focused less on diagnostic assessment and more on adverse effects of social media use and psychiatric comorbidities. Additionally, many studies focus on broad concepts such as "internet addiction" and fail to look specifically at social media use. Prevalence rates vary wildly from 2.8% in Nigerian [57] to 47% in Malaysian [58] college students due to a lack of consensus on psychometric assessment and likely cultural/technological differences across countries as well. However, the six-item Bergen Social Media Addiction scale has been most widely studied across multiple countries [59–61] and found to be valid and reliable across periods of three months in China [62].

As with other technological addictions, it is likely more clinically helpful to focus on associated symptoms and psychosocial factors that can precipitate and predispose adolescents to excessive social media use. A systematic review examining social media addiction and attachment style discovered a significant positive association between insecure attachment (anxious and avoidant) and dysfunctional social media use [63]. They posit that those with insecure attachment appear to use social media as a way of compensating for a lack of affection from family and peers. Montserrat and colleagues opted to conceptualize social media addiction as a multidimensional construct and concluded that gender and physical attractiveness seems to be the most relevant predictors of social media use [64]. They found that younger adolescent females with a physically attractive body image and a disinhibited, neurotic, and extraverted personality tend to use social media more often. Additionally, they report that narcissism is the most influential factor in the prediction of "nomophobia," a colloquial term to describe fear of being detached from one's mobile phone connectivity.

Despite (limited) qualitative research showing that adolescents themselves even perceive social media as a threat to mental well-being [65], experts are careful not to over-pathologize social media use given the immense benefits of online communities for children and adolescents.

Pornography

Adolescent pornography consumption has been a focus of moral panic for years despite a growing body of research to explore the topic. Since 2016, US state legislatures have passed resolutions declaring pornography a public health crisis. However, a systematic review of studies during the year 2000–2017 showed that research trends in this field have focused primarily on individual factors such as development, victimization, mental health, and religiosity, while ignoring contextual and activity-related factors to adolescent pornography use [66]. For example, large disparities in prevalence rates are highly likely due to differences in cultural attitudes toward sex, not just between countries but even within culturally diverse cities such as New York City. One study of 433 adolescents in New York City reporting that about 55% of adolescents visit pornographic websites [67] and another study of 529 Greek adolescents reported 20% of teenagers visit pornographic websites and about half of this group visit these sites on a regular basis [68].

Though the DSM does not give any guidance regarding addiction to pornography specifically, it has introduced Hypersexual Disorder (HD) with the publication of DSM-5. In contrast to substance-use disorders, gambling disorder, and internet gaming disorder (see section on Symptomatology and Controversy), HD requires 80% of symptom endorsement to meet criteria for diagnosis. Additionally, Criterion D excludes adolescents under age 18. The WHO also introduced Compulsive sexual behavior disorder (CSBD) with the release of ICD-11, which does not specify an age limit [69]:

Compulsive sexual behaviour disorder is characterised by a persistent pattern of failure to control intense, repetitive sexual impulses or urges resulting in repetitive sexual behaviour. Symptoms may include repetitive sexual activities becoming a central focus of the person's life to the point of neglecting health and personal care or other interests, activities and responsibilities; numerous unsuccessful efforts to significantly reduce repetitive sexual behaviour; and continued repetitive sexual behaviour despite adverse consequences or deriving little or no satisfaction from it. The pattern of failure to control intense, sexual impulses or urges and resulting repetitive sexual behaviour is manifested over an extended period of time (e.g., 6 months or more), and causes marked distress or significant impairment in personal, family, social, educational, occupational, or other important areas of functioning. Distress that is entirely related to moral judgments and disapproval about sexual impulses, urges, or behaviours is not sufficient to meet this requirement.

Objectively, pornography use does appear to be linked to concerning attitudinal and behavioral outcomes [70]. It has been associated with greater casual sexual behavior, greater sexual objectification of partners, greater risk of sexual aggression, more permissive views of sex, and more stereotypical beliefs about gender roles [71]. However, the potential benefits of adolescent pornography use from sexual to mental health have not been examined as closely. There is some evidence that adolescents, especially sexual minorities, may use pornography as a way to explore their sexuality in a private, nonjudgmental, and safe setting [72], similar to the arguments for the benefits of video game use outlined above.

Researchers from Boston University developed and implemented a pornography literacy class for high school students to improve their knowledge, attitudes, and behavioral intentions related to pornography, healthy relationships, and sexual consent [73]. The program consists of nine 60-min sessions and aims to train adolescents to become peer-facilitators for subsequent groups. The intervention appeared to clarify knowledge related to the legality of minors viewing porn and sending sexually explicit photos of themselves to other minors, which is legal and illegal, respectively. Participants in the program were also less likely to view pornography as a helpful way to learn about sex and changed their perceptions surrounding violent and derogatory sexual behaviors [74]. As of June 2017, only 24 states and the District of Columbia mandate sex education be provided to students in public school and only 13 states require that the instruction be medically accurate [75].

Video Streaming

Since video streaming and video-on-demand (VOD) services did not become widely available until the mid-2000s, there is very little research on the topic of streaming addiction or "binge-watching" as it is referred to in the literature, and even less research focused on adolescents. The first systematic review of the evidence base was published in January 2020 and concluded that binge-watching remains an ill-defined construct with no consensus on its operationalization or measurement [76]. Similarly to IGD, researchers agree that there can exist high levels of nonproblematic binge-watching and avoidance of over-pathologization is key.

However, the literature does emphasize that binge-watching is likely an emotion-focused coping strategy [77] and stress certain demographics, motivations, personality traits, and harmful outcomes for clinicians to be aware of. Unfortunately, associations with gender, age, and education level are largely inconclusive; however, single individuals are generally more severe binge-watchers than those in romantic partnerships [78]. The motivations behind binge-watching were found to be compensatory in nature, including passing time, dealing with loneliness, and escape from everyday worries [79]. Additionally, binge-watchers were found to be characterized by insecure attachment [80], low agreeableness, conscientiousness, and openness, and high levels of neuroticism [81]. Above all, researchers emphasize the impulsive nature and predilection toward immediate gratification of binge-watchers [82, 83]. One study showed that binge-watching frequency was associated with reduced sleep quality, daytime fatigue, and insomnia, with cognitive presleep arousal mediating those relationships [84], and another study supported these dangerous outcomes by negatively correlating healthy diet with overall binge-watching [85]. That being said, several studies also convey that binge-watching imbues a healthy sense of perceived autonomy [86] and harmonious passion [81]. However, outcomes such as stronger parasocial (one-sided) relationships with protagonists [87] make it difficult to draw positive conclusions about the associations with higher narrative transportation, media enjoyment, and media effects on beliefs, emotions, and behaviors [88].

Based on the evidence, it seems likely that binge-watching is less likely to be as clinically problematic as other forms of media consumption given that artistic visual media are simply not designed to be as addictive as video games, pornography, or social media.

Case

Patient's name has been changed and all information de-identified

Paulo is a 13-year-old male with past diagnoses of attention-deficit/hyperactivity disorder (ADHD), oppositional defiant disorder, and conduct disorder who presented with his mother to a psychiatric emergency room in the middle of the night after a verbal and physical altercation in the context of his mother attempting to set limits around his video game playing. He specifically plays online multiplayer games until late into the night, which causes his mother to become frustrated and concerned about his health. His mother reports that he otherwise does well academically in school and has had no behavioral issues while in class. Paulo has a history of witnessing domestic violence between mother and romantic partner. His father has been incarcerated since his birth. Family history is significant for his mother being diagnosed with "schizophrenia and bipolar disorder." She had been in outpatient treatment, but stopped recently.

Per chart review and history taking, Paulo was in psychiatric treatment in another state within the year prior to presentation for excessive internet gaming, aggressive behavior, and sleep deprivation, which was helpful until his mother's romantic partner convinced him to withdraw from treatment. Paulo and his mother subsequently moved and have visited local emergency rooms four times in the six months prior to presentation for aggressive and oppositional behavior in the context of his mother setting limits on his video game playing. Paulo was evaluated again, diagnosed with ADHD and adjustment disorder, and prescribed six weeks worth of methylphenidate and guanfacine. Paulo eventually refused to follow up for therapy or medication management, but agreed to take the medication he was already prescribed. He was not seen in a psychiatric emergency room for exactly eight weeks after he was evaluated and prescribed medication.

Case Discussion

As Paulo was seen in an emergency setting, his case offers only a snapshot of his symptomatology and course of treatment. However, there are several helpful clinical pearls that we can draw from his history.

While Paulo clearly carries diagnoses that would directly explain his externalizing behaviors, he also has a trauma history that includes witnessing domestic violence between caregivers and disrupted attachment from his father. These factors may also contribute to Paulo's ongoing behaviors via mood symptoms (depressed mood, irritability, social withdrawal) that are known mediators and contributors to the development of IGD. Given that no known classroom-based assessments of Paulo's ADHD exist and he and his mother both denied any academic or behavioral issues in school, his diagnosis of ADHD is questionable. However, during the time that he was being prescribed a stimulant and an alpha-agonist, he was not brought to an emergency room for behavioral reasons, which was a clear shift from the usual pattern seen on chart review.

Paulo's case emphasizes the multifactorial impact of underlying comorbidities, traumatic experiences, and parental-child relations on the severity and frequency of internet gaming. Though he was not formally assessed for IGD on presentation, his history behooves us to consider IGD as a diagnosis. Furthermore, while we cannot be sure what symptoms improved while taking these medications due to Paulo's refusal to follow up with care, his lack of need for emergency services during this time coupled with the evidence that methylphenidate can improve IGD symptoms is encouraging for the use of medication to improve outcomes for children with IGD.

Conclusion

While the internet has become such an integral part of all of our lives, online gaming in particular plays such a large role in the lives of adolescents today that many teachers have begun to "gamify" their curricula by turning to online tools such as *Kahoot* in the hopes of engaging their students. Some researchers have mixed feelings about this approach, wondering what message having a "gamified" curriculum sends to children who might be at risk of developing IGD and urge schools to provide education to parents on recognizing potentially problematic behavior [89].

That being said, it is important to note that some video games provide a constant and random stream of rewards, while others provide them more judiciously and purposefully, such as part of the progression of a storyline. These differences in the nature of gameplay can drastically influence dopamine release and either encourage or inhibit addictive behavior [53]. For example, the first FDA-approved video game for the behavioral treatment of ADHD (named EndeavorRx) involves repetitive levels requiring focused eye movements and discernment tasks that fluctuate in difficulty and provide rewards based on the user's performance. EndeavorRx simulates the Test of Variables of Attention (TOVA) task in a fun and engaging way and has been shown to objectively improve measures of inattention, but not hyperactivity, in children with ADHD [90]. Thus, gamifying educational curricula may be potentially advantageous for children with undiagnosed or untreated ADHD due to parental reservations about medications or other comorbidities masking the diagnosis.

Based on the lack of guidelines or consensus on diagnosis and management of technological addictions, it is clear that experts remain judicious about over-pathologizing such widely used and relatively novel media.

Recommendations for Clinicians

Based on the evidence reviewed in this chapter, it appears pertinent that screening for internet-based addictions become a routine preventative measure as electronic media becomes more ubiquitous and easy for children to access. More specifically, IGD screening during a psychiatric intake may improve diagnostic clarity, enhance outcomes, and increase rapport with children and adolescents. However, it is also important to educate parents on the diagnosis and encourage them to avoid stigmatizing the use of electronic media in the home, which can lead to parent-child relational issues and worsen comorbid psychiatric conditions. When the use of medication is warranted, the use of SSRIs, bupropion, and stimulants can improve IGD symptoms safely depending on symptomatology and comorbid diagnoses.

Multiple Choice Questions
1. When considered together, which features of problematic gaming increase the likelihood of an IGD diagnosis the most?
   A. Preoccupation and negative consequences
   B. Withdrawal and loss of control
   C. Preoccupation and withdrawal
   D. Loss of control and preoccupation
   Correct Answer: B
2. Which two factors were noted to be predictors of persistence of high-risk IGD status in adolescents?
   A. Depressive symptoms and ADHD symptoms
   B. Playing over 120 min of online games per day and ADHD symptoms
   C. Poor attachment to parents and depressive symptoms
   D. Playing over 240 min of online games per day and ADHD symptoms
   Correct Answer: D
3. Which of the following medications was proven to have greater efficacy over another medication for reduction in IGD symptoms?
   A. Escitalopram
   B. Methylphenidate
   C. Bupropion
   D. Atomoxetine
   Correct Answer: C

References

1. Stevens MW, Dorstyn D, Delfabbro PH, King DL. Global prevalence of gaming disorder: A systematic review and meta-analysis. Aust N Z J Psychiatry. 2021;55(6):553–68. https://doi.org/10.1177/0004867420962851.
2. Fam JY. Prevalence of internet gaming disorder in adolescents: A meta-analysis across three decades. Scand J Psychol. 2018;59(5):524–31. https://doi.org/10.1111/sjop.12459.
3. Paulus FW, Ohmann S, von Gontard A, Popow C. Internet gaming disorder in children and adolescents: a systematic review. Dev Med Child Neurol. 2018;60(7):645–59. https://doi.org/10.1111/dmcn.13754.
4. Kristensen JH, Pallesen S, King DL, Hysing M, Erevik EK. Problematic gaming and sleep: a systematic review and meta-analysis. Front Psychiatry. 2021;12:675237. https://doi.org/10.3389/fpsyt.2021.675237.
5. Block JJ. Issues for DSM-V: internet addiction. Am J Psychiatry. 2008;165(3):306–7. https://doi.org/10.1176/appi.ajp.2007.07101556.
6. Goh B. Three hours a week: Play time's over for China's young video gamers. Reuters2021.

7. Young KS. Internet addiction: the emergence of a new clinical disorder. 104th annual meeting of the American Psychological Association. Toronto, Canada; 1996.
8. Markey PM, Ferguson CJ. Internet gaming addiction: disorder or moral panic? Am J Psychiatry. 2017;174(3):195–6. https://doi.org/10.1176/appi.ajp.2016.16121341.
9. Przybylski AK, Weinstein N, Murayama K. Internet gaming disorder: investigating the clinical relevance of a new phenomenon. Am J Psychiatry. 2017;174(3):230–6. https://doi.org/10.1176/appi.ajp.2016.16020224.
10. King DL, Haagsma MC, Delfabbro PH, Gradisar M, Griffiths MD. Toward a consensus definition of pathological video-gaming: a systematic review of psychometric assessment tools. Clin Psychol Rev. 2013;33(3):331–42. https://doi.org/10.1016/j.cpr.2013.01.002.
11. Pontes HM, Schivinski B, Brzozowska-Wos M, Stavropoulos V. Laxer clinical criteria for gaming disorder may hinder future efforts to devise an efficient diagnostic approach: a tree-based model study. J Clin Med. 2019;8(10). https://doi.org/10.3390/jcm8101730.
12. Charlton JP. A factor-analytic investigation of computer 'addiction' and engagement. Br J Psychol. 2002;93(Pt 3):329–44.
13. Charlton JP, Danforth IDW. Distinguishing addiction and high engagement in the context of online game playing. Comput Hum Behav. 2007;23(3):1531–48. https://doi.org/10.1016/j.chb.2005.07.002.
14. Pontes HM, Kiraly O, Demetrovics Z, Griffiths MD. The conceptualisation and measurement of DSM-5 Internet Gaming Disorder: the development of the IGD-20 Test. PLoS One. 2014;9(10):e110137. https://doi.org/10.1371/journal.pone.0110137.
15. Brunborg GS, Hanss D, Mentzoni RA, Pallesen S. Core and peripheral criteria of video game addiction in the game addiction scale for adolescents. Cyberpsychol Behav Soc Netw. 2015;18(5):280–5. https://doi.org/10.1089/cyber.2014.0509.
16. Fuster H, Carbonell X, Pontes HM, Griffiths MD. Spanish validation of the Internet Gaming Disorder-20 (IGD-20) Test. Comput Hum Behav. 2016;56:215–24.
17. Snodgrass JG, Zhao W, Lacy MG, Zhang S, Tate R. Distinguishing core from peripheral psychiatric symptoms: addictive and problematic internet gaming in North America, Europe, and China. Cult Med Psychiatry. 2019;43(2):181–210. https://doi.org/10.1007/s11013-018-9608-5.
18. Organization WH: ICD-11: Gaming Disorder. https://icd.who.int/browse11/l-m/en#/http://id.who.int/icd/entity/338347362. Accessed 4 Jan 2022.
19. Jeong H, Yim HW, Jo SJ, Lee SY, Kim E, Son HJ, et al. Study protocol of the internet user cohort for unbiased recognition of gaming disorder in early adolescence (iCURE), Korea, 2015-2019. BMJ Open. 2017;7(10):e018350. https://doi.org/10.1136/bmjopen-2017-018350.
20. Jeong H, Yim HW, Lee S-Y, Lee HK, Potenza MN, Kwon J-H, et al. Discordance between self-report and clinical diagnosis of Internet gaming disorder in adolescents. Scientific Reports. 2018;8(1):1–8.
21. King DL, Chamberlain SR, Carragher N, Billieux J, Stein D, Mueller K, et al. Screening and assessment tools for gaming disorder: A comprehensive systematic review. Clin Psychol Rev. 2020;77:101831. https://doi.org/10.1016/j.cpr.2020.101831.
22. Jo SJ, Jeong H, Son HJ, Lee HK, Lee SY, Kweon YS, et al. Diagnostic usefulness of an ultra-brief screener to identify risk of online gaming disorder for children and adolescents. Psychiatry Investig. 2020;17(8):762–8. https://doi.org/10.30773/pi.2019.0279.
23. Hygen BW, Skalicka V, Stenseng F, Belsky J, Steinsbekk S, Wichstrom L. The co-occurrence between symptoms of internet gaming disorder and psychiatric disorders in childhood and adolescence: prospective relations or common causes? J Child Psychol Psychiatry. 2020;61(8):890–8. https://doi.org/10.1111/jcpp.13289.
24. Jeong H, Yim HW, Lee SY, Lee HK, Potenza MN, Lee H. Factors associated with severity, incidence or persistence of internet gaming disorder in children and adolescents: a 2-year longitudinal study. Addiction. 2021;116(7):1828–38. https://doi.org/10.1111/add.15366.
25. Strittmatter E, Kaess M, Parzer P, Fischer G, Carli V, Hoven CW, et al. Pathological Internet use among adolescents: comparing gamers and non-gamers. Psychiatry Res. 2015;228(1):128–35. https://doi.org/10.1016/j.psychres.2015.04.029.

26. Tian Y, Yu C, Lin S, Lu J, Liu Y, Zhang W. Sensation seeking, deviant peer affiliation, and internet gaming addiction among chinese adolescents: the moderating effect of parental knowledge. Front Psychol. 2018;9:2727. https://doi.org/10.3389/fpsyg.2018.02727.

27. Kwon JH, Chung CS, Lee J. The effects of escape from self and interpersonal relationship on the pathological use of Internet games. Community Ment Health J. 2011;47(1):113–21. https://doi.org/10.1007/s10597-009-9236-1.

28. Beranuy M, Carbonell X, Griffiths MD. A qualitative analysis of online gaming addicts in treatment. Int J Mental Health Addiction. 2013;11(2):149–61.

29. Wichstrom L, Stenseng F, Belsky J, von Soest T, Hygen BW. Symptoms of internet gaming disorder in youth: predictors and comorbidity. J Abnorm Child Psychol. 2019;47(1):71–83. https://doi.org/10.1007/s10802-018-0422-x.

30. Hwang H, Hong J, Kim SM, Han DH. The correlation between family relationships and brain activity within the reward circuit in adolescents with Internet gaming disorder. Sci Rep. 2020;10(1):9951. https://doi.org/10.1038/s41598-020-66535-3.

31. Han DH, Bae S, Hong J, Kim SM, Son YD, Renshaw P. Resting-state fMRI study of ADHD and internet gaming disorder. J Atten Disord. 2021;25(8):1080–95. https://doi.org/10.1177/1087054719883022.

32. Zajac K, Ginley MK, Chang R, Petry NM. Treatments for Internet gaming disorder and Internet addiction: a systematic review. Psychol Addict Behav. 2017;31(8):979–94. https://doi.org/10.1037/adb0000315.

33. Han DH, Hwang JW, Renshaw PF. Bupropion sustained release treatment decreases craving for video games and cue-induced brain activity in patients with Internet video game addiction. Exp Clin Psychopharmacol. 2010;18(4):297–304. https://doi.org/10.1037/a0020023.

34. Bae S, Hong JS, Kim SM, Han DH. Bupropion shows different effects on brain functional connectivity in patients with internet-based gambling disorder and internet gaming disorder. Front Psychiatry. 2018;9:130.

35. Nam B, Bae S, Kim SM, Hong JS, Han DH. Comparing the effects of bupropion and escitalopram on excessive internet game play in patients with major depressive disorder. Clin Psychopharmacol Neurosci. 2017;15(4):361–8. https://doi.org/10.9758/cpn.2017.15.4.361.

36. Wolfling K, Muller KW, Dreier M, Ruckes C, Deuster O, Batra A, et al. Efficacy of short-term treatment of internet and computer game addiction: a randomized clinical trial. JAMA Psychiatry. 2019;76(10):1018–25. https://doi.org/10.1001/jamapsychiatry.2019.1676.

37. Song J, Park JH, Han DH, Roh S, Son JH, Choi TY, et al. Comparative study of the effects of bupropion and escitalopram on Internet gaming disorder. Psychiatry Clin Neurosci. 2016;70(11):527–35. https://doi.org/10.1111/pcn.12429.

38. Han DH, Lee YS, Na C, Ahn JY, Chung US, Daniels MA, et al. The effect of methylphenidate on Internet video game play in children with attention-deficit/hyperactivity disorder. Compr Psychiatry. 2009;50(3):251–6. https://doi.org/10.1016/j.comppsych.2008.08.011.

39. Park JH, Lee YS, Sohn JH, Han DH. Effectiveness of atomoxetine and methylphenidate for problematic online gaming in adolescents with attention deficit hyperactivity disorder. Hum Psychopharmacol. 2016;31(6):427–32. https://doi.org/10.1002/hup.2559.

40. Yao Y-W, Chen P-R, Chiang-shan RL, Hare TA, Li S, Zhang J-T, et al. Combined reality therapy and mindfulness meditation decrease intertemporal decisional impulsivity in young adults with Internet gaming disorder. Computers in Human Behavior. 2017;68:210–6.

41. Gonzalez-Bueso V, Santamaria JJ, Fernandez D, Merino L, Montero E, Jimenez-Murcia S, et al. Internet gaming disorder in adolescents: personality, psychopathology and evaluation of a psychological intervention combined with parent psychoeducation. Front Psychol. 2018;9:787. https://doi.org/10.3389/fpsyg.2018.00787.

42. Torres-Rodriguez A, Griffiths MD, Carbonell X, Oberst U. Treatment efficacy of a specialized psychotherapy program for Internet Gaming Disorder. J Behav Addict. 2018;7(4):939–52. https://doi.org/10.1556/2006.7.2018.111.

43. Li H, Wang S. The role of cognitive distortion in online game addiction among Chinese adolescents. Children Youth Services Rev. 2013;35(9):1468–75.

44. Park SY, Kim SM, Roh S, Soh MA, Lee SH, Kim H, et al. The effects of a virtual reality treatment program for online gaming addiction. Comput Methods Programs Biomed. 2016;129:99–108. https://doi.org/10.1016/j.cmpb.2016.01.015.
45. Li W, Garland EL, McGovern P, O'Brien JE, Tronnier C, Howard MO. Mindfulness-oriented recovery enhancement for internet gaming disorder in US adults: a stage I randomized controlled trial. Psychol Addictive Behav. 2017;31(4):393.
46. Kim SM, Han DH, Lee YS, Renshaw PF. Combined cognitive behavioral therapy and bupropion for the treatment of problematic on-line game play in adolescents with major depressive disorder. Comput Human Behav. 2012;28(5):1954–9.
47. Han DH, Kim SM, Lee YS, Renshaw PF. The effect of family therapy on the changes in the severity of on-line game play and brain activity in adolescents with on-line game addiction. Psychiatry Res. 2012;202(2):126–31. https://doi.org/10.1016/j.pscychresns.2012.02.011.
48. Sakuma H, Mihara S, Nakayama H, Miura K, Kitayuguchi T, Maezono M, et al. Treatment with the Self-Discovery Camp (SDiC) improves Internet gaming disorder. Addict Behav. 2017;64:357–62. https://doi.org/10.1016/j.addbeh.2016.06.013.
49. Pornnoppadol C, Ratta-apha W, Chanpen S, Wattananond S, Dumrongrungruang N, Thongchoi K, et al. A comparative study of psychosocial interventions for internet gaming disorder among adolescents aged 13–17 years. Int J Mental Health Addiction. 2020;18(4):932–48.
50. Cragg A, Taylor C, Toombs B. Video games: Research to improve understanding of what players enjoy about video games, and to explain their preferences for particular games. London: British Board of Film Classification; 2007. p. 1–107.
51. Olson CK. Children's motivations for video game play in the context of normal development. Rev General Psychol. 2010;14(2):180–7.
52. Jansz J. The emotional appeal of violent video games for adolescent males. Commun Theory. 2005;15(3):219–41.
53. Weigle PE, Englander EK. "My kid's always online, but what can I do about it?" helping families manage media. J Am Acad Child Adolescent Psychiatry. 2021;60(10):S39.
54. Keles B, McCrae N, Grealish A. A systematic review: the influence of social media on depression, anxiety and psychological distress in adolescents. Int J Adolescence Youth. 2020;25(1):79–93.
55. Saul JS, Rodgers RF. Adolescent eating disorder risk and the online world. Child Adolesc Psychiatr Clin N Am. 2018;27(2):221–8. https://doi.org/10.1016/j.chc.2017.11.011.
56. Wilksch SM, O'Shea A, Ho P, Byrne S, Wade TD. The relationship between social media use and disordered eating in young adolescents. Int J Eating Disorders. 2020;53(1):96–106.
57. Olowu AO, Seri FO. A study of social network addiction among youths in Nigeria. J Social Sci Policy Rev. 2012;4(1):63–71.
58. Jafarkarimi H, Sim ATH, Saadatdoost R, Hee JM. Facebook addiction among Malaysian students. Int J Information Educ Technol. 2016;6(6):465.
59. Monacis L, de Palo V, Griffiths MD, Sinatra M. Social networking addiction, attachment style, and validation of the Italian version of the Bergen Social Media Addiction Scale. J Behav Addict. 2017;6(2):178–86. https://doi.org/10.1556/2006.6.2017.023.
60. Dadiotis A, Bacopoulou F, Kokka I, Vlachakis D, Chrousos GP, Darviri C, et al. Validation of the Greek version of the Bergen Social Media Addiction Scale in undergraduate students. EMBnet J. 2021:26. https://doi.org/10.14806/ej.26.1.975.
61. Stanculescu E. The Bergen Social Media Addiction Scale validity in a Romanian sample using item response theory and network analysis. Int J Ment Health Addict 2022:1–18. https://doi.org/10.1007/s11469-021-00732-7.
62. Chen IH, Strong C, Lin YC, Tsai MC, Leung H, Lin CY, et al. Time invariance of three ultrabrief internet-related instruments: Smartphone Application-Based Addiction Scale (SABAS), Bergen Social Media Addiction Scale (BSMAS), and the nine-item Internet Gaming Disorder Scale- Short Form (IGDS-SF9) (Study Part B). Addict Behav. 2020;101:105960. https://doi.org/10.1016/j.addbeh.2019.04.018.

63. D'Arienzo MC, Boursier V, Griffiths MD. Addiction to social media and attachment styles: a systematic literature review. Int J Mental Health Addiction. 2019;17(4):1094–118.
64. Peris M, de la Barrera U, Schoeps K, Montoya-Castilla I. Psychological risk factors that predict social networking and internet addiction in adolescents. Int J Environ Res Public Health. 2020;17(12):4598.
65. O'Reilly M, Dogra N, Whiteman N, Hughes J, Eruyar S, Reilly P. Is social media bad for mental health and wellbeing? Exploring the perspectives of adolescents. Clin Child Psychol Psychiatry. 2018;23(4):601–13.
66. Alexandraki K, Stavropoulos V, Anderson E, Latifi MQ, Gomez R. Adolescent pornography use: a systematic literature review of research trends 2000-2017. Curr Psychiatry Rev. 2018;14(1):47–58.
67. Braun-Courville DK, Rojas M. Exposure to sexually explicit Web sites and adolescent sexual attitudes and behaviors. J Adolesc Health. 2009;45(2):156–62. https://doi.org/10.1016/j.jadohealth.2008.12.004.
68. Tsitsika A, Critselis E, Kormas G, Konstantoulaki E, Constantopoulos A, Kafetzis D. Adolescent pornographic internet site use: a multivariate regression analysis of the predictive factors of use and psychosocial implications. Cyberpsychol Behav. 2009;12(5):545–50. https://doi.org/10.1089/cpb.2008.0346.
69. Organization WH: ICD-11: Compulsive sexual behavior disorder. https://icd.who.int/browse11/l-m/en#/http%3a%2f%2fid.who.int%2ficd%2fentity%2f1630268048. Accessed 30 Jan 2022.
70. Grubbs JB, Kraus SW. Pornography use and psychological science. a call for consideration Curr Directions Psychol Sci. 2021;30(1):68–75.
71. Peter J, Valkenburg PM. Adolescents and pornography: a review of 20 years of research. J Sex Res. 2016;53(4-5):509–31. https://doi.org/10.1080/00224499.2016.1143441.
72. Bőthe B, Vaillancourt-Morel M-P, Bergeron S, Demetrovics Z. Problematic and non-problematic pornography use among LGBTQ adolescents: a systematic literature review. Curr Addiction Rep. 2019;6(4):478–94.
73. Rothman EF, Daley N, Alder J. A pornography literacy program for adolescents. Am J Public Health. 2020;110(2):154–6. https://doi.org/10.2105/AJPH.2019.305468.
74. Rothman EF, Adhia A, Christensen TT, Paruk J, Alder J, Daley N. A pornography literacy class for youth: Results of a feasibility and efficacy pilot study. Am J Sexuality Educ. 2018;13(1):1–17.
75. Institute TG: State laws and policies: Sex and HIV education. https://www.guttmacher.org/state-policy/explore/sex-and-hiv-education; 2017. Accessed.
76. Flayelle M, Maurage P, Di Lorenzo KR, Vögele C, Gainsbury SM, Billieux J. Binge-watching: what do we know so far? A first systematic review of the evidence. Curr Addiction Reports. 2020;7(1):44–60.
77. Flayelle M, Canale N, Vögele C, Karila L, Maurage P, Billieux J. Assessing binge-watching behaviors: Development and validation of the "Watching TV Series Motives" and "Binge-watching Engagement and Symptoms" questionnaires. Comput Human Behav. 2019;90:26–36.
78. Ahmed AA-AM. New era of TV-watching behavior: binge watching and its psychological effects. Media Watch. 2017;8(2):192–207.
79. Starosta J, Izydorczyk B, Lizyńczyk S. Characteristics of people's binge-watching behavior in the "entering into early adulthood" period of life. Health Psychol Report. 2019;7(2)
80. Tukachinsky R, Eyal K. The psychology of marathon television viewing: antecedents and viewer involvement. Mass Commun Society. 2018;21(3):275–95.
81. Toth-Kiraly I, Bothe B, Toth-Faber E, Haga G, Orosz G. Connected to TV series: quantifying series watching engagement. J Behav Addict. 2017;6(4):472–89. https://doi.org/10.1556/2006.6.2017.083.
82. Riddle K, Peebles A, Davis C, Xu F, Schroeder E. The addictive potential of television binge watching: Comparing intentional and unintentional binges. Psychol Popular Media Culture. 2018;7(4):589.

83. Shim H, Lim S, Jung EE, Shin E. I hate binge-watching but I can't help doing it: the moderating effect of immediate gratification and need for cognition on binge-watching attitude-behavior relation. Telematics Informatics. 2018;35(7):1971–9.
84. Exelmans L, Van den Bulck J. Binge viewing, sleep, and the role of pre-sleep arousal. J Clin Sleep Med. 2017;13(8):1001–8. https://doi.org/10.5664/jcsm.6704.
85. Spruance L, Karmakar M, Kruger J, Vaterlaus J. "Are you still watching?": correlations between binge TV watching, diet and physical activity. J Obesity Weight Manag. 2017;
86. Granow VC, Reinecke L, Ziegele M. Binge-watching and psychological well-being: media use between lack of control and perceived autonomy. Commun Res Reports. 2018;35(5):392–401.
87. Erickson SE, Dal Cin S, Byl H. An experimental examination of binge watching and narrative engagement. Social Sci. 2019;8(1):19.
88. Green MC, Brock TC, Kaufman GF. Understanding media enjoyment: the role of transportation into narrative worlds. Commun Theory. 2004;14(4):311–27.
89. Gentile DA, Bailey K, Bavelier D, Brockmyer JF, Cash H, Coyne SM, et al. Internet gaming disorder in children and adolescents. Pediatrics. 2017;140(Suppl 2):S81–S5. https://doi.org/10.1542/peds.2016-1758H.
90. Kollins SH, DeLoss DJ, Canadas E, Lutz J, Findling RL, Keefe RSE, et al. A novel digital intervention for actively reducing severity of paediatric ADHD (STARS-ADHD): a randomised controlled trial. Lancet Digit Health. 2020;2(4):e168–e78. https://doi.org/10.1016/S2589-7500(20)30017-0.

Peer-to-Peer Support and the Strength of Online Communities

9

Alexandra Hamlyn and Pantea Farahmand

Introduction

More than half of children and adolescents report going online several times a day, and roughly one-fourth of teens report being online "almost constantly." Though there are many reasons young people may want to spend their time online, social networking has been identified as a popular activity for most. Online social networking has been celebrated and vilified for its impact on childhood development. Headlines have emerged criticizing online communities, gaming sites, and social media for increasing youth access to graphic and violent content, setting unrealistic social and beauty standards, reducing in vivo socialization, and putting children at risk for being bullied or exploited. Despite the risks, the digital age continues to expand globally, and more children are going online every day. Online socialization has evolved rapidly including email, bulletin board messages, real-time chats, blogs and microblogs (i.e., twitter), social media sites, photo-share, visual pin boards, serial short video stories, live streams, and more. Novel technologies including iPhones, telephone applications, and smart watches have emerged to permit easy access to online communities. New career concepts such as influencers, social media marketers/managers, and online reputation builders have also emerged. In this chapter, we explore how the internet offers children and adolescents peer-to-peer support and a sense of belonging through online communities. We also discuss recommendations for safeguarding underage users from the potential dangers of online socialization [1–4].

A. Hamlyn (✉) · P. Farahmand
Department of Child and Adolescent Psychiatry, NYU Child Study Center, NYU Grossman, School of Medicine, New York, NY, USA
e-mail: Alexandra.hamlyn@nyulangone.org; Pantea.farahmand@nyulangone.org

© The Author(s), under exclusive license to Springer Nature Switzerland AG 2023
A. Spaniardi, J. M. Avari (eds.), *Teens, Screens, and Social Connection*,
https://doi.org/10.1007/978-3-031-24804-7_9

The Impact of Social Media on Adolescent Mental Health on Neurotypical Kids

Social media can have positive and negative effects on children and adolescents; however, the negative effects often seem to gain more attention than the benefits. That being said, when social media use among young adults was compared to negative outcomes such as anxiety, overall mental health, and loneliness, results demonstrated that social media use was a poor predictor for any of these issues. Even more, social media use among youth can help individuals significantly [5].

The obvious benefit of social media use among adolescents is the ability to form an online friendship or community with people from anywhere in the world. This in turn increases diversity and allows adolescents to find others who share their same ideas and interests. Adolescents may feel more connected to others, less lonely, and gain more confidence in themselves. Social media can also help adolescents gain knowledge in areas they may otherwise not be exposed to, such as politics, current events, economy, etc. [6].

Social media also creates an outlet for people to express themselves in their online community without the fear of rejection or embarrassment they may receive during face-to-face interactions. For example, if someone has a passion for writing short stories, but was always embarrassed and unsure of themselves, they could post this online with anonymity, and put their creations out into the world. Overall, social media and online communities provide adolescents with a space where they can feel more comfortable being themselves than they might otherwise in their in-person communities.

Benefits of Social Media During Challenging Universal Experiences

Children and adolescents heavily rely on social contact and peer relationships on a regular basis for mood stabilization, validation, brain development, and personal growth. Certain circumstances such as natural disasters, pandemics, and war can greatly impact the ability for individuals to have face-to-face interactions. The COVID-19 pandemic had a great impact on socialization of all age groups as lockdowns took place around the world, and people were told to keep distance from others and reduce physical contact. This lead to increased feelings of loneliness, isolation, depression, and anxiety—specifically in children and adolescents as they often exceedingly depend on peer support [7].

Social media can be an exceptional resource during these situations as this can allow adolescents the ability to find social connections that they are not able to seek out in the community. In fact, adolescents that use social media as a way to be more social with peers reported that they felt more connected to peers and were able to rely on these connections for increased support during challenging circumstances. Adolescents that feel they have adequate social support during crises are able to cope better than adolescents that do not have the same increased social support [8]. The ability to be socially connected to friends and family through different online communities likely increases this social support and leads to increased happiness and better coping skills during a crisis like the COVID-19 pandemic. Another added benefit is that adolescents were also able to engage with a more diverse population that may not be available in their community. Furthermore, studies have demonstrated being active on social media and engaging with others by commenting or posting on their own social media actually improves well-being [8].

In addition to making social connections over social media, individuals were also able to seek out more information about the current events during the COVID-19 pandemic using social media. The ability to access information regarding the pandemic and being able to feel more prepared and up to date on situations has a tremendous impact on adolescents' well-being. The awareness of the pandemic and possibility of becoming more prepared actually demonstrated the ability to help individuals better self-regulate their mood. The capability of having access to this information via social media is something that was not as prominent prior to the internet and greatly helped adolescents during this current pandemic [7].

How Social Media Can Help Kids with Mood and Anxiety Disorders

Social media's effect on adolescents with diagnosed mood and anxiety disorders can range. While some studies have demonstrated that it can increase symptoms of these disorders, it is important to note that social media can also help provide a sense of support and belonging in this population. Adolescents with mental illness have reported multiple benefits from social media by being able to interact with peers online. Social media platforms allow adolescents to share their own mental health journey and feel a greater connection to others who may also be living with mental health conditions. The ability to connect with others with similar experiences is an opportunity that these individuals may not experience in their day-to-day life in the community [9]. Subsequently, this can reduce symptoms of anxiety and depression as the individual may not feel alone. Even more, these adolescents can discuss their mental health without the stigma these individuals may face in the community. Adolescents who are able to learn to speak comfortably about this may then feel more empowered to break the stigma that mental health conditions still hold [9].

Adolescents have also reported that they have been able to learn more about their mental health and gain insight into their illness and symptoms through these online communities. Additionally, these individuals learn how to seek help and learn different coping skills to use on a regular basis to help manage their depression or anxiety. Adolescents who have specific questions about their illness or symptoms that ask friends online are likely to gain emotional support as well as informational support from others who have experienced something similar [9]. This is a different response than adolescents may get if they ask friends in the community who have not experienced what the individual is experiencing. These adolescents then feel more empowered when seeking help and can even be more knowledgeable and able to ask appropriate questions with less intimidation while speaking about mental health [9]. This could provide a decrease in symptoms and give the adolescent hope for the future that they will be able to grow and reach their full potential.

Social Media and Kids with Developmental Disabilities and Movement Disorders

Children and adolescents with developmental disabilities and movement disorders (such as tic disorders) often have a harder time than other children assimilating into social situations. This is due to a variety of reasons consisting of stigmatization, bullying, and social exclusion. In addition to having a difficult time socializing, finding providers that specialize in these fields can be challenging for the child and the caregivers. Social media can offer a multitude of benefits in this population ranging from support groups to better understanding their condition [10].

Online communities are helpful for gaining more insight and information regarding certain developmental disabilities and movement disorders. Online groups can be particularly helpful as you do not always have to be in a specific geographical location and can find more peers with similar disorders. Some have reported that they were able to find better care while talking to online communities as specialists can be hard to find. Another added benefit is that individuals who were not actively seeking help were explained the benefits of speaking to a professional and were able to schedule appropriate appointments [10]. Online communities can also help individuals learn different coping skills and ways to handle their disability on a day-to-day basis.

Social media for adolescents with developmental disabilities and movement disorders can greatly impact socialization. This population often faces many barriers to socializing in person, and social media can provide outlets for these individuals to find a safe space with peers who are facing similar stigmatization [10]. This can allow the individual to feel more connected and empowered thus decreasing feelings of loneliness. This support can be more beneficial than in person situations as there are less geographical restrictions, which then allows individuals to find more peers from all over the globe. This lessens financial demands as caregivers do not have to pay to travel and find in-person support groups and communities. Studies have demonstrated that individuals that use online support for movement disorders felt less isolated because they were able to form friendships online and had greater feelings of belonging to a community. Individuals also stated they had more confidence and had hope for a better future. These individuals felt more empowered to speak out against discrimination and negative stigma about movement disorders [10].

Social Media Benefits for Underrepresentative Populations

The LGBTQ+ population may spend more time on social media than the non-LGBTQ+ population for a variety of reasons. There is still a significant amount of stigma surrounding the LGBTQ+ community and online communities. Online communities can help LGBTQ+ adolescents explore their identity in a safe space with individuals who also are exploring their sexuality. This time spent on social media may allow these adolescents to feel more connected to peers and feel less isolated [11].

Online communities for the LGBTQ+ population can help provide emotional support for adolescents while they are still questioning their sexuality and help them find information they may not find in their community. Studies have suggested that using social media actually increased coping and sense of well-being in this population by feeling less isolated and gaining emotional support. Additionally, websites that allowed individuals to be creative with their content helped adolescents design images of youth that may not be common in current media. This then allowed the user to feel more validated in their observation of themself [11].

Similar to the LGBTQ+ community, other minority groups such as Black or Latinx adolescents also find social media to be a place where they can find peers with similar views and experiences and gain support. Additionally, Black and Latinx youth were found to create more media for social networking sites than their white or Asian counterparts, allowing them to have an outlet to voice their opinions and gain support from others who share their beliefs [12].

Advantages of Online Gaming Communities

Adolescents spend a significant amount of time playing video games and, for some, this is an escape from the real world. For adolescents that feel they have a hard time fitting in with peers at school or in their community, online gaming communities can help them feel welcomed and create a friend group for these individuals.

When people think of video games, a lot of people think of violent, aggressive, competitive games where you are playing against an opponent. Violent video games are often thought to be associated with increased aggression and violence in real life; however, data is mixed as to if there is actually a correlation between the two. Playing any type of video game, including violent games, has demonstrated that gaming can promote prosocial behavior and increase general well-being [13]. These online communities can promote effective communication, helpful behaviors, and ability to cooperate as part of a team. Adolescents who play multiplayer games or games with civic experiences feel more confident to speak out about other social and civic movements in their life outside of gaming [14].

Online gaming communities can also be a significant resource for children who may not feel comfortable in their own skin or have trouble making friends in the real world. Children who are not comfortable with certain aspects of themselves may allow themselves to experiment with different genders, looks, and sexuality online.

One study demonstrated that people who played video games felt more comfortable in the gaming environment as they were not judged for their appearance, gender, or sexuality. In addition to feeling more comfortable in regards to appearance, people who made friends online stated that they felt more confident speaking to these friends about topics they would otherwise not feel as comfortable speaking about in their day-to-day lives [15].

The Influence of Social Media on Online Political Activism

As stated earlier, social media can be a place where adolescents gain information about current events and politics. This can also be a place where youth can start to form their own opinions and find their voice to speak about what they feel passionate about or what they think about the state of the world. Many adolescents have admitted to obtaining information regarding the 2020 election through social media websites such as YouTube, Instagram, TikTok, and Facebook [16]. However, adolescents are not just gaining information from these websites, but they are actively posting and discussing these topics on social media as well. Tufts Medical Center found that over half of the youth were found to have engaged in creating media about politics or current social issues. Creating content on social media was also found to have positive effects. The youth that did engage in creating content surrounding politics and social issues stated they felt more empowered when in person and also felt their voices were heard and that their voices mattered. Adolescents gaining access and learning about political and social issues at a young age may help more adolescents become interested in these topics [16].

Recommendations to Parents

It is important to always monitor what content your child is engaging with on social media and online communities. Different social media groups or websites can provide a host of resources and support depending on what the youth is looking to gain from these communities. Helping a teen safely navigate social media by explaining the risks but also the benefits is imperative. Parents should help the youth find safe spaces and monitor the communities to ensure they are engaging properly. Additionally, being involved in what adolescents are creating and posting on social media can also be helpful for parents when monitoring their child's social media presence.

Case Study

Katherine is a 16-year-old female who has never struggled with psychiatric illness before. She previously had a large group of friends but has recently moved with her family from another state and attends in-person high school. She is in 10th grade and feels like she does not have a lot of friends at school as she had to start in the middle of the academic year. Katherine now feels anxious prior to the school day, and she often reports headaches and feeling nauseous most weekday mornings. Luckily, Katherine has been able to keep in touch with her friends from her previous school through social media. She feels this helps her feel more connected to them. Katherine has been expressing her feelings about her new school to her mother, and her mother was able to look up online support groups for children who have recently moved. Katherine joined this online support group and recognized that many teenagers struggle emotionally when moving to a new place. Katherine was even able to identify someone from her current school, Samantha, in this support group. Katherine and her mother reached out to Samantha and her family through social media. Samantha's family was very receptive and set up a time for Katherine and Samantha to meet outside of the support group. Katherine and Samantha became friends and Samantha introduced Katherine to her friends at their new school. Katherine no longer feels sick in the morning, and she looks forward to going to school so that she can see her new friends.

Conclusion

Today's children and adolescents are spending more and more time online, and with the constant emergence of new social media websites, it appears the time spent on these websites will only increase. It is impossible to discuss social media without reporting the potential negative effects of spending so much time online. It is also imperative that we explore all of the benefits these children and adolescents can gain from spending time on these websites. The online communities that adolescents can participate in while visiting these websites not only help them feel part of a community and engage with other peers, but this engagement also increases wellness [8]. Social media can particularly help adolescents who are already struggling with pre-existing mental health disorders like anxiety, depression, or tic disorders [9, 10]. Individuals with mental health disorders can use these online communities to find peers who have previously or are currently experiencing similar struggles. These adolescents are able to gain insight and support from these peers and feel more knowledgeable and confident about their current disorder [9].

Social networking and different websites also provide adolescents with information and knowledge about politics, social dilemmas, and world news [6]. Not only does social media help inform today's youth about these topics, but individuals now have a platform where they can speak about these topics and feel that their voices are heard. When adolescents feel empowered like this, they also will feel more comfortable speaking about these topics in their day-to-day experiences and likely carry over this confidence into other aspects of their lives [16].

Overall, social media and online communities can offer a host of benefits that are not often spoken about when discussing children and adolescents and the internet. It is vital that we include this information when discussing social media as these online communities can be exceptionally supportive for youth. Online communities can help youth find peers that have similar experiences and feel connected to others during different stages of their life.

Multiple Choice Questions

1. Social media can be helpful for adolescents during challenging universal experiences in what way?
    A. Social media can allow adolescents the ability to find social connections if they are not able to seek conditions in the community.
    B. Having social support online can allow adolescents to cope better with the experience.
    C. Social media may allow adolescents to seek out more information and feel better prepared, which in turn helps the individual to better regulate their mood.
    D. All of the above.
    Correct Answer: D
2. How is the online gaming community beneficial to adolescents?
    A. Promotes violent behavior in adolescents.
    B. Allows children to experiment with different genders, looks, and sexuality.
    C. Can lead to addiction in adolescents that is more beneficial than substances.
    D. The gaming community is not helpful to adolescents in any way.
    Correct Answer: B
3. How can caregivers help their children navigate the internet?
    A. By explaining risks and benefits of different websites.
    B. By monitoring the different communities and websites the child visits.
    C. There is no way to safely navigate the internet and social media.
    D. Answers A and B.
    Correct Answer: D

References

1. Arnett JJ. Adolescents' uses of media for self-socialization. J Youth Adolesc [Internet]. 1995;24(5):519–33. https://doi.org/10.1007/bf01537054.
2. Stornaiuolo A. Commentary on Zizek. Hum Dev [Internet]. 2017;60(5):233–8. https://www.jstor.org/stable/26765176
3. UNICEF Office of Research-Innocenti. Global Kids Online Comparative Report [Internet]. UNICEF-IRC. [cited 2022 Feb 14]. https://www.unicef-irc.org/publications/1059-global-kids-online-comparative-report.html
4. US NSF—NSF and the birth of the internet [Internet]. Nsf.gov. [cited 2022 Feb 8]. https://www.nsf.gov/news/special_reports/nsf-net/index.jsp
5. Berryman C, Ferguson CJ, Negy C. Social media use and mental health among young adults. Psychiatr Q [Internet]. 2018;89(2):307–14. [cited 2022 Feb 7]. https://pubmed.ncbi.nlm.nih.gov/29090428/

6. Rawath S, Satheeshkumar R, Kumar V. A study on impact of social media on youth. J Manag [Internet]. 2019;6(1). [cited 2022 Feb 7]. https://papers.ssrn.com/abstract=3526175

7. Cauberghe V, Van Wesenbeeck I, De Jans S, Hudders L, Ponnet K. How adolescents use social media to cope with feelings of loneliness and anxiety during COVID-19 lockdown. Cyberpsychol Behav Soc Netw [Internet]. 2021;24(4):250–7. https://doi.org/10.1089/cyber.2020.0478.

8. Orben A, Tomova L, Blakemore S-J. The effects of social deprivation on adolescent development and mental health. Lancet Child Adolesc Health [Internet]. 2020;4(8):634–40. https://doi.org/10.1016/S2352-4642(20)30186-3.

9. Prescott J, Hanley T, Ujhelyi K. Peer communication in online mental health forums for young people: directional and nondirectional support. JMIR Ment Health [Internet]. 2017;4(3):e29. https://doi.org/10.2196/mental.6921.

10. Perkins V, Coulson NS, Davies EB. Using online support communities for Tourette syndrome and tic disorders: online survey of users' experiences. J Med Internet Res [Internet]. 2020;22(11):e18099. https://doi.org/10.2196/18099.

11. Craig SL, Eaton AD, McInroy LB, Leung VWY, Krishnan S. Can social media participation enhance LGBTQ+ youth well-being? Development of the social media benefits scale. Soc Media Soc [Internet]. 2021;7(1):205630512198893. https://doi.org/10.1177/2056305121988931.

12. Young people created media to uplift their voices in 2020 [Internet]. Tufts.edu. [cited 2022 Feb 7]. https://circle.tufts.edu/latest-research/young-people-created-media-uplift-their-voices-2020

13. Halbrook YJ, O'Donnell AT, Msetfi RM. When and how video games can be good: a review of the positive effects of video games on well-being. Perspect Psychol Sci [Internet]. 2019;14(6):1096–104. https://doi.org/10.1177/1745691619863807.

14. Granic I, Lobel A, Engels RCME. The benefits of playing video games. Am Psychol [Internet]. 2014;69(1):66–78. https://doi.org/10.1037/a0034857.

15. Cole H, Griffiths MD. Social interactions in massively multiplayer online role-playing gamers. Cyberpsychol Behav [Internet]. 2007;10(4):575–83. https://doi.org/10.1089/cpb.2007.9988.

16. Young people turn to online political engagement during COVID-19 [Internet]. Tufts.edu. [cited 2022 Feb 14]. https://circle.tufts.edu/latest-research/young-people-turn-online-political-engagement-during-covid-19

Internet Safety: Family and Clinician Protection of Kids Online

10

Renee C. Saenger and Anna H. Rosen

Introduction

The internet is a relatively new phenomenon, and yet, it has radically altered the landscape of childhood and adolescence. Children are spending more time than ever on the Internet, social media, user-created content, video games, mobile applications (apps), virtual or augmented reality, and Internet-connected toys [1]. According to the 2019 U.S. Department of Commerce American Community Survey, 95% of children ages three and older have access to the internet at home via computer-based or smartphone access [2]. Concerns about internet safety and supervision now start at birth with World Health Organization guidelines that recommend against any screen time in the first year of life [3]. Over one-third of parents of children under 12 believe that their children started to interact with a smartphone before they were 5 years old [4]. Internet safety as a broad category that includes not just screen time, but also cyberbullying and social media, online sexual exploitation, digital advertising, adult-oriented content, and gaming.

The first federal law to address internet safety for children was passed by Congress and signed into law by President Bill Clinton in 1998. The Children's Online Privacy Protection Act, or COPPA, effective April 21, 2000, was as in response to the growth of electronic commerce (e-commerce) and collection of personal data from children under 13 years old [5]. COPPA requires that websites operating from the United States or under US jurisdiction and/or appeal to children under 13 years old require parental approval before collecting data from children. As such, COPPA outlines for website operators specific expectations including

---

R. C. Saenger (✉) · A. H. Rosen
Department of Child and Adolescent Psychiatry, New York Presbyterian-Weill Cornell
Medical College, New York, NY, USA
e-mail: rcs7001@med.cornell.edu; ash9006@med.cornell.edu

© The Author(s), under exclusive license to Springer Nature Switzerland AG 2023
A. Spaniardi, J. M. Avari (eds.), *Teens, Screens, and Social Connection*,
https://doi.org/10.1007/978-3-031-24804-7_10

145

privacy policies as well as when and how to seek verifiable consent from a parent or guardian, and what responsibilities a website operator must protect children's privacy and safety online including restrictions on the marketing to those under 13. Revisions to COPPA in 2013 placed time limits on data retention and collection [6]. COPPA regulations also apply to third parties who can access a child's information.

The FTC is explicit that the goals of COPPA are to place parents in control over what information is collected from their children online [7]. To this end, COPPA legislation does not limit content offered to children, nor does it prevent children from lying about their age to access content. The question of access to internet content for children was in part addressed with Congress' passage of the Children's Internet Protection Act (CIPA) in 2000 [8]. CIPA's legislation is specifically tied to three agencies: the Federal Communications Commission (FCC), the Department of Education (D. of Ed.), and the Institute of Museum and Library Services (IMLS), all of whom receive internet access or internal connections through the E-rate program [9]. The E-rate program offers discounts for telecommunications, internet access, and internal connections for eligible schools and libraries, according poverty level and support to rural districts. In early 2001, the FCC issued rules implementing CIPA and provided updates to those rules in 2011 [10].

Federal legislation sets some content limits upon organizations that use federal funding to support internet related costs. Yet the legislation makes clear that the task of supervising children's screen time and internet exposure largely falls on parents [11]. In a recent survey, 61% of parents endorsed asking a doctor or medical professional on parenting advice related to screen time [4]. Protecting children from the digital environment requires a multipronged approach that involves parents, educators, clinicians, policymakers, and regulatory/design solutions. In response to the changing environment and heightened concerns for safety of children, over the last ten years, the American Academy of Pediatrics (AAP) and the American Academy of Child and Adolescent Psychiatry (AACAP) have published policy statements on internet safety to guide parents and clinicians [11–16].

The Role of Parents

An understanding of the technology is essential for parents to engage with children on the topic of "digital literacy" and safety. The term "digital literacy" refers to the knowledge that families need in order to create a safe and effective relationship with the digital world that is at all our fingertips [11]. This involves an ongoing dialogue between parents and children so that everyone can stay on top of new developments, devices, functionality, policies, and regulations. Children are more likely than adults to have an "interpersonal" approach to technology in which they are more trusting and less comprehending of the commercialization of content [17]. Moreover, considering socioeconomic backgrounds and disparities in knowledge about the digital world is important for understanding children's attitudes toward online safety.

Children often feel a sense of mastery over technology and may be less inclined to ask parents "who don't understand" [18].

The AAP recommends that parents "know what their children are downloading." Supervision of children's access to online content can be enhanced with the use of privacy settings on personal devices and social media. The AAP promotes a family media plan to help parents set limits around screen time for each child and ensure adequate sleep, physical activity, and time away from media [16]. Parents should talk to their children about advertising on the internet and be explicit about the self-interested intentions of businesses who embed their advertisements in user content. Most importantly, parents should engage their children in questioning the content on the internet and critically analyze features that encourage certain behaviors (targeted advertising, autoplay that keeps children watching longer, solicitation of personal information). Parents should ensure that both they and their children understand the details of their privacy settings and have ongoing conversations about online citizenship and safety [11, 19]. [See Table 10.1 for internet safety education online programs designed for kids]

Parent-child collaboration around internet usage (i.e., discussions around cyberbullying, encouraging critical viewing, and co-usage of content, apps, and games) are referred to by the AAP as "active parental mediation practices." Another broad category of parental practices surrounding internet usage is defined by the AAP as "restrictive mediation." Restrictive methods include rules around media/screen use including time and content limits [19]. Restrictive mediation also includes e-Discipline or the common parental practice of rewarding good behavior with additional screen time and conversely taking away screen time as a consequence for negative behaviors. Interestingly, one study showed that e-Discipline may inadvertently have the opposite effect and increase children's total daily screen time [20]. Other studies have suggested that active restriction of children's media usage should begin from a very early age and include limits on duration (including all devices), content, timing (not before bedtime), eating habits, and peer involvement [21]. Only a handful of studies have investigated the longitudinal effects of differing parenting practices on children's media usage. Furthermore, parental involvement changes as children develop. Parents may initially use more active restriction for younger children and then graduate to a more collaborative and active approach with adolescents [19]. See Table 10.2 for a list of AACAP recommendations for parents.

Table 10.1 Helpful Resources for Parents

https://www.childrenscommissioner.gov.uk/digital/who-knows-what-about-me/
https://www.consumerreports.org/digital-security/online-security-and-privacy-guide/
https://www.commonsensemedia.org/privacy-and-internet-safety
https://www.healthychildren.org/English/media/Pages/default.aspx
https://www.ted.com/talks/sonia_livingstone_parenting_in_the_digital_age/
transcript?language=en

Table 10.2 AACAP recommendations for parents [13]

Limit the amount of time a child spends on screens.

Teach a child that talking to "screen names" in a chat room or on games is the same as talking to strangers.

Teach a child never to give out any personal identifying information to an individual or website.

Teach a child to never agree to actually meet someone they have met online.

Never give a child credit card numbers or passwords that will enable online purchases or access to inappropriate services or sites.

Remind a child that not everything they see or read online is true.

Make use of parental control features so as to restrict access to inappropriate content.

Provide an individual e-mail address only if a child is mature enough to manage it, and plan to periodically monitor the child's e-mail.

Monitor the content of a child's social media accounts and personal websites.

Teach a child to use the same courtesy in communicating with others online as they would if speaking in person.

Insist that a child follow the same guidelines at other computers/devices they may have access to such as those at school, libraries, or friends' homes.

The Role of Clinicians

Clinicians can be instrumental in helping parents mediate their children's media usage and promote internet safety. Like parents, clinicians must also improve their own digital literacy by taking the time to understand the myriad of apps, platforms, and smart devices that exist. An informed clinician can in turn help parents mediate their children's media usage in a developmentally appropriate way. Routinely asking about media usage and family rules around media is essential. A clinician can assist in the development of a family media plan that sets reasonable and consistent limits around screen usage. For example, it is recommended that children of all ages should not sleep with devices in their bedrooms and should avoid screen use one hour before bedtime [15]. Clinicians can help parents become more attuned to internet safety by reminding parents of the importance of both monitoring and speaking to their children about topics including privacy, advertising, disturbing content, and excessive usage [16]. Clinicians can educate parents about the link between screen time and obesity and the negative effects of media use on sleep and school performance [22]. Studies have shown that earlier exposure of adolescents to sexual behaviors, substance use, and alcohol on the internet is associated with earlier onset of these behaviors [11, 23]. Teenagers are increasingly drawn to "influencers" on social media that promote eating disordered behaviors, self-injury, and suicide [24]. Clinicians can also help parents model good media usage. Studies have shown that parents who watch more television are more likely to have children who watch more television [25]. More recently, it was shown that parents who turn to a mobile device while with a young child are less likely to engage the child in conversation; it is unclear what long-term effect this could have on a child's development [21]. However, clinicians must be careful not to overemphasize the negative aspects of online media. Parents can be encouraged to emphasize the opportunities to connect, co-view, and create that the internet and technology at large offers [19]. Finally, clinicians can work with schools, educators, and policy makers to help design digital literacy programs for children of all socioeconomic backgrounds and provide online resources to parents.

Pediatric providers (including pediatricians, child and adolescent psychiatrists, child and adolescent psychologists and social workers) are uniquely situated to advise families on specific areas of concern involving internet safety. They can also help identify young people who are spending too much time online and developing a maladaptive relationship with the internet. Problematic internet use (PIU) is defined as internet use that is risky, excessive, or impulsive in nature, leading to adverse life consequences, specifically physical, emotional, social or functional impairment. Associated consequences of PIU include conduct problems, hyperactivity, symptoms of depression, difficulty with daily functions and physical health, trouble concentrating, suicidal ideation, and poor interpersonal relationships [26]. Adolescents (especially males) who experience family dissatisfaction and who have parents with mental health issues are more likely to become overly reliant on the internet for mood regulation and relationships. Other studies have shown that mental health disorders at large are risk factors for developing an overuse disorder. Although traditionally thought of as internet gaming disorder, it has become clear that internet overuse can include other online nongaming activities [27]. The Problematic and Risky Internet Use Screening Scale (PRIUSS) is an 18-item scale validated for use in pediatric populations [28]. Whereas the AAP used to recommend strict limits on hours of "screen time" per day, newer evidence suggests that time spent online is not the only factor at play in PIU. Rather, PIU is closely connected to adolescent depression, feelings of alienation, a "need to belong," and narcissistic character traits [26]. Programs developed to target PIU in children include psychoeducation about the dangers of overuse, self-control techniques, limit-setting and time management skills, and alternative activities. The most successful programs include a broad mental health approach and address family factors and parent training [29]. There are scant evidence-based screening tools and interventions to identify and address PIU and further research is needed in this area [30].

Clinicians can also help to identify children who are the perpetrators and victims of cyberbullying as well as provide parenting support in this area. They can remind parents that the transition to middle school is a critical window to manage the risks of cyberbullying because of the increased use of screens in conjunction with a developmental (and possibly sociological) propensity toward offline bullying that occurs in this age group with peak cyberbullying occurring at ages 13–15 [31]. Cyberbullying may have a particularly injurious emotional impact on youth due to the seeming permanent nature of online postings, the possibility of increased hostile content that anonymity provides, and the intrusive nature of postings that can happen any time of day or night [32, 33]. Strategies for reducing cyberbullying include improving parent-child communication, increased parental monitoring of technology use, and increased parental support/warmth [31]. A 2018 study found that parental discussion and higher levels of connective co-use were more effective in reducing cyberbullying risk than restrictive practices such as rigid time limits or rules regarding what type of media children are allowed to use [34]. Another recent study found a significant association between authoritative parenting practices (high parental involvement, high strictness/supervision, high autonomy granting) and low online victimization among teens. Clinicians can help address parent-child relational difficulties that may be contributing to a child's reluctance to approach a parent for help with these issues [35]. Screening measures and questions related to youth violence can be routinely utilized by clinicians to uncover both online and offline aggression as it is well substantiated that most cyberbullying occurs in conjunction with offline bullying [27]. Helping parents find online resources can also be a helpful part of supporting parents' efforts to provide coping strategies to their children. Finally, clinicians can foster communication by serving as important liaisons between parents and schools given that cyberbullying occurs most often in the context of adolescent school peer relationships.

Sexual exploitation of minors online, sexual content on the internet, and sexting represent a significant area of concern for parents and families. Clinicians can provide education on these topics and engage adolescents in open conversations about sex and relationships [36]. Although parents are often most concerned about strangers targeting their children online, most adults who solicit children online were acquaintances from offline contexts [37]. In fact, there is significant overlap and similarity between internet-mediated and more typical forms of child sexual abuse. Rather than simply warning children "to never meet up with someone you meet online," a better approach would be to encourage youth to make better decisions surrounding romantic relationships and sex. Influencing teen sexual behaviors has always been difficult since teenagers have a developmental interest in exploring romance, relationships, and sexual activity. Sexting, or the passing of sexual images or messages via mobile devices or the internet, is not necessarily problematic if consensual, but can become risky if images are obtained via coercion or pressure or are shared without consent [27, 38]. Abusive sexting, termed "aggravated sexting" in the literature, can be distinguished from the sexting that occurs between consenting peers [37]. A clinician can help parents separate moral and reputational concerns from sexting that is malicious and exploitative. There is scant evidence to support the use of scare tactics with teens such as warnings about the proliferation of images on the internet and the potential future consequences of future opportunities (i.e., college, jobs, relationships). Again, helping parents communicate with their children more broadly about sex, relationships, and personal boundaries has shown to be the most effective means of altering risky behaviors [39].

Clinicians must also be aware of the content surrounding suicide and self-harm behaviors that exists on the internet. There has been increasing concern about websites that specifically guide and encourage youth to engage in suicide, suicidal behaviors, and self-harm behaviors including eating disordered behaviors. Adolescents who are depressed, anxious, and prone to risk-taking [27] behaviors are particularly drawn to this content. At-risk youth may feel supported when they engage in chat-room discussions though the coping skills encouraged are often dangerous and maladaptive [27]. Child mental health clinicians play an essential role in identifying and treating these children. Online interest in self-harm and suicide has been associated with internet overuse and cyberbullying, but has its roots in offline contributors including mental health disorders, family relational issues, trauma histories, and social/peer challenges [40]. This area of internet safety is more broadly included in youth suicide and self-harm prevention. Clinicians must involve parents and families in psychoeducation and treatment, provide alternate coping skills and therapies, and liaise with schools [41]. Clinicians who work in schools (i.e., school psychologists and social workers) may be in a unique position to provide essential school-based screenings to identify vulnerable children [42]. Finally, it is important to appreciate that the internet may have both an aggravating and mitigating impact on young people who are seeking mental health support [43]. Clinicians who work in pediatrics, mental health, and within schools should be aware of the online influence on vulnerable children in the larger context of a general promotion of youth suicide and self-harm awareness and prevention.

It is increasingly essential for clinicians to be aware of unsafe and problematic internet related practices among children and adolescents. Yet previous studies have shown that over 50% of pediatric mental health professionals felt ill equipped to manage such concerns [44]. Similarly, parents often feel unable to monitor and advise their children on issues involving internet safety. Intergenerational dynamics may play a role. Further research is necessary to evaluate the effectiveness of the current safeguards [26].

The following two cases elaborate on the indications, risks, and benefits related to online safety and ways in which internet usage and access have come to clinical attention.

Case 1 Aja is a 16-year-old heterosexual female living with her parents in a suburban area. She is the youngest of four siblings and, according to the patient and her parents, has received the least supervision in "all teenage things." Aja does very well in school. She is a star athlete and hopes to study at a premiere college with the stated goal "to become president." She initially presented to an outpatient psychiatrist with complaints of anxiety and depression. She described herself as more isolated from friends, even as covid precautions were lifted and she and her friends were vaccinated. Treatment included Cognitive Behavioral Therapy (CBT) and the start of an SSRI antidepressant medication, which led to remission of symptoms. Together, Aja and her psychiatrist decided to space out sessions to once a month. Over the summer, Aja worked at a supermarket and met her first boyfriend. She was excited to share this with her psychiatrist and waited until the end of a session to ask if it was true that her parents could be investigated for inappropriate pictures on her phone (which was part of her parents' phone plan). The patient explained that her friend told her that her parents could go to jail if she was sending pictures to her boyfriend. The patient was concerned. She liked sending the pictures and said they were not nude, but often taken on her own. She thought of the pictures as artistic expressions and appreciated the glowing responses from her boyfriend.

Aja was reaching out to a trusted adult. Her psychiatrist made space in their session to learn about Aja's experience, "everyone is doing it" and "I like sending these pictures to him." With that said, she appreciated that the psychiatrist took the time to explore the content of the photos, to establish that sending pictures that were clothed, even if they were somewhat suggestive, abstract, and/or artistic, was not an example of coercive sexual content. Together, they explored their meaning to the patient, trying to understand if there were other ways to create that experience without creating a digital footprint that existed on someone's else's phone. The psychiatrist was able to orient the patient to the laws around exchange of sexual content from a minor, the potential implications for her parents and for herself. Treatment could then focus on ways to facilitate the positive experience around her sexuality and her connection to her boyfriend while engaging in behaviors with less risk.

Case 2 Raymond is a 9-year-old male with psychiatric diagnosis of ADHD-combined type. He receives care from a psychiatrist to address hyperactivity, organization, social skills and his parents are engaged in Parent Management Training with a psychologist. Raymond's family history is significant for major depressive disorder, substance-use disorders, and bipolar disorder. Both of Raymond's parents relied upon Raymond's engagement with his tablet during the months of lockdown for covid-19. Raymond was the calmest and seemed the most content when he was engaged with video games. This was a relief to Raymond's parents who were concerned about the impact so much time at home would have upon Raymond and his siblings. Several months into covid, Raymond's parents reached out to their son's psychiatrist concerned that their son was developing paranoid ideation. The patient's father revealed that he overheard their son speaking to someone named Susan and when he asked Raymond about Susan, Raymond would frequently mumble to himself, dismiss his parent's comments, and once divulged, "she is out to get me."

During the psychiatrists' next meeting with Raymond, he asked him about his gaming and asked him to share some of his gaming during the session. Raymond, eager to show off his gaming skills and have additional screen time shared his device with his doctor and pointed out that one of the characters in the game, named Susan was frequently "following" him. Raymond's psychiatrist reality tested with Raymond, "Was Susan real?" he probed, "No, she's a robot in a video game, " Raymond bemused. He did add however that she frequently followed him, and as it became clear to the psychiatrist this was in fact part of the point of the game. During this session, Raymond's psychiatrist remained curious about Raymond's online life—had he made friends with other people? (no); did he let others join his gaming? (no); did he give his name and address to other players? (no). In his screening questions, it became clear that Raymond was not paranoid, but was involved with a very lively online world without his parent's understanding and supervision. Raymond's psychiatrist wondered if Raymond could invite his parents to play with him, to get a sense of the game, and to screen for any suspicious invitations before he was permitted to play independently. This struck Raymond's psychiatrist as the right balance of making Raymond's experience less isolated from his parents and offering an opportunity for his parents to observe and then enter this important part of his world.

Conclusion

These case examples highlight the complex interplay between technology, aspects of development including childhood imaginary play and adolescent exploration of sexuality and relationships, and role of parenting and clinician guidance. Also present is the increased reliance on screens due to the covid-19 pandemic. An overarching theme in the above cases as well as in the treatment of youth generally is the therapeutic alliance that forms between treating clinicians and families. It is the bridge to facilitate open, honest, and nonjudgmental conversations.

Navigating children and adolescent's online life is a nascent role both for parents and clinicians. Parents and clinicians must remain vigilant in their digital literacy and clinicians should tend to internet safety in their anticipatory guidance with parents. There is evidence to support the role of beginning conversations at children's early well visits and as a part of any psychiatric and/or psychological evaluation. It is incumbent upon parents to anticipate that their children will need supervision and scaffolding around screen time and internet use. Clinicians must maintain a non-judgmental and informed position with a keen awareness of the developmental and psychiatric issues tied to internet use and children's safety. We encourage clinicians to remain available for education, reflection, and recommendations for parents and their families.

Multiple Choice Questions
1. What year was the first federal law to address internet safety for children passed?
   A. 1990
   B. 1998
   C. 2001
   D. 2015
   Correct Answer: B
2. What does the term "digital literacy" refer to?
   A. Being able to understand all the acronyms and slang used on social media
   B. The knowledge needed to create a safe and effective relationship to the digital world
   C. Learning how to program and create websites and smartphone applications
   Correct Answer: B
3. What is the most important approach a clinician can take when talking to young people about their internet use?
   A. Nonjudgmental and inquisitive
   B. Punitive and accusatory
   C. Avoidance of direct questions
   D. Use cautionary tales and scare tactics
   Correct Answer: A

References

1. Moreno MA, Egan KG, Bare K, Young HN, Cox ED. Internet safety education for youth: stakeholder perspectives. BMC Public Health. 2013;13(1):1–6.
2. Irwin V, Zhang J, Wang X, Hein S, Wang K, Roberts A, York C, Barmer A, Bullock Mann F, Dilig R, Parker S. Report on the condition of education 2021 (NCES 2021-144). U.S. Department of Education. Washington, DC: National Center for Education Statistics; 2021. https://nces.ed.gov/pubsearch/pubsinfo.asp?pubid=2021144. Accessed 31 Jan 22.
3. World Health Organization. Guidelines on physical activity, sedentary behaviour and sleep for children under 5 years of age. World Health Organization; 2019. https://apps.who.int/iris/handle/10665/311664. License: CC BY-NC-SA 3.0 IGO.
4. Pew Research Center, July 2020, "Parenting children in the age of screens."
5. The Children's Online Privacy Protection Act of 1998 (COPPA) is a United States federal law, located at 15 U.S.C. §§ 6501–6506 (Pub. L. 105–277 (text) (PDF), 112 Stat.
6. Children's Online Privacy Protection Rule (COPPA), 15 U.S.C. § 6501-6508; 2013.
7. FTC guide: Children's Internet Protection Act. Federal Trade Commission; April 2013. https://www.ftc.gov/tips-advice/business-center/guidance/childrens-online-privacy-protection-rule-not-just-kids-sites. Accessed 31 Jan 22.
8. Children's Internet Protection Act (CIPA), 20 U.S.C. § 9134; 2000.
9. FCC guide: Children's Internet Protection Act. Federal Communications Commission; December 2019. https://www.fcc.gov/sites/default/files/childrens_internet_protection_act_cipa.pdf. Accessed 31 Jan 22.
10. Children's Internet Protection Act (CIPA), 47 U.S.C. § 254; 2011.
11. Radesky J, Chassiakos YLR, Ameenuddin N, Navsaria D. Digital advertising to children. Pediatrics. 2020;146(1)
12. AACAP Facts for Families No. 54, "Screen Time and Children"; February 2020.
13. AACAP Facts for Families No. 59, "Internet Use in Children"; 2015.
14. AACAP Facts for Families No. 100, "Social Media and Teens"; 2018.
15. Croke LM. Use of media by school-aged children and adolescents: a policy statement from the AAP. Am Fam Phys. 2017;96(1):56–7.
16. AAP Council on Communications and Media, & MBE. Media use in school-aged children and adolescents. Pediatrics. 2016;138(5):e20162592.
17. Stoilova M, Livingstone S, Nandagiri R. Digital by default: children's capacity to understand and manage online data and privacy. Media and Communication; 2020.
18. Livingstone S, Stoilova M, Nandagiri R. Children's data and privacy online: growing up in a digital age: an evidence review. London: London School of Economics and Political Science; 2019.
19. Coyne SM, Radesky J, Collier KM, Gentile DA, Linder JR, Nathanson AI, et al. Parenting and digital media. Pediatrics. 2017;140(Supplement 2):S112–6.
20. Hawi NS, Rupert MS Impact of e-Discipline on children's screen time. Cyberpsychology, Behavior, and Social Networking, 2015;18(6):337–342.
21. AAP Council on Communications and Media. Media and young minds. Pediatrics. 2016;138(5):e20162591.
22. De Jong E, Visscher TLS, HiraSing RA, Heymans MW, Seidell JC, Renders CM. Association between TV viewing, computer use and overweight, determinants and competing activities of screen time in 4-to 13-year-old children. Int J Obes. 2013;37(1):47–53.
23. Quigley J. Alcohol Use by Youth. Pediatrics. 2019;144(1):e20191356–e20191356.
24. Marchant A, Hawton K, Stewart A, Montgomery P, Singaravelu V, Lloyd K, et al. A systematic review of the relationship between internet use, self-harm and suicidal behaviour in young people: the good, the bad and the unknown. PLoS One. 2017;12(8):e0181722.
25. Bleakley Amy, Amy B Jordan, and Michael Hennessy. "The Relationship between Parents' and Children's Television Viewing." Pediatrics (Evanston) 132.2(2013):E364–371. Web.
26. D'Angelo J, Moreno MA. Screening for problematic internet use. Pediatrics. 2020;145(Supplement 2):S181–5.

27. Finkelhor D, Walsh K, Jones L, Mitchell K, Collier A. Youth internet safety education: aligning programs with the evidence base. Trauma Violence Abuse. 2020:1524838020916257.
28. Jelenchick LA, Eickhoff J, Christakis DA, Brown RL, Zhang C, Benson M, Moreno MA. The Problematic and Risky Internet Use Screening Scale (PRIUSS) for adolescents and young adults: scale development and refinement. Comput Human Behav. 2014;35:171–8.
29. Schneider LA, King DL, Delfabbro PH. Family factors in adolescent problematic Internet gaming: A systematic review. J Behav Addictions. 2017;6(3):321–33.
30. King DL, Delfabbro PH, Doh YY, Wu AM, Kuss DJ, Pallesen S, et al. Policy and prevention approaches for disordered and hazardous gaming and Internet use: An international perspective. Prevent Sci. 2018;19(2):233–49.
31. Helfrich EL, Doty JL, Su YW, Yourell JL, Gabrielli J. Parental views on preventing and minimizing negative effects of cyberbullying. Children Youth Serv Rev. 2020;118:105377.
32. Duke NN, Borowsky IW. Adolescent interpersonal violence: implications for health care professionals. Primary Care Clin Off Pract. 2014;41(3):671–89.
33. Fu KW, Chan CH, Ip P. Exploring the relationship between cyberbullying and unnatural child death: an ecological study of twenty-four European countries. BMC Pediatr. 2014;14(1):1–6.
34. Padilla-Walker LM, Coyne SM, Kroff SL, Memmott-Elison MK. The protective role of parental media monitoring style from early to late adolescence. J Youth Adolescence. 2018;47(2):445–59.
35. Marengo N, Borraccino A, Charrier L, Berchialla P, Dalmasso P, Caputo M, Lemma P. Cyberbullying and problematic social media use: an insight into the positive role of social support in adolescents—data from the Health Behaviour in School-aged Children study in Italy. Public Health. 2021;199:46–50.
36. Madigan S, Villani V, Azzopardi C, Laut D, Smith T, Temple JR, et al. The prevalence of unwanted online sexual exposure and solicitation among youth: a meta-analysis. J Adolescent Health. 2018;63(2):133–41.
37. Mitchell KJ, Jones LM, Finkelhor D, Wolak J. Trends in unwanted online experiences and sexting. Durham, NH: Crimes against Children Research Center; 2014.
38. Van Ouytsel J, Lu Y, Ponnet K, Walrave M, Temple JR. Longitudinal associations between sexting, cyberbullying, and bullying among adolescents: Cross-lagged panel analysis. J Adolescence. 2019;73:36–41.
39. Livingstone S, Smith PK. Annual research review: harms experienced by child users of online and mobile technologies: the nature, prevalence and management of sexual and aggressive risks in the digital age. J Child Psychol Psychiatry. 2014;55(6):635–54.
40. Görzig A. Adolescents' viewing of suicide-related web content and psychological problems: differentiating the roles of cyberbullying involvement. Cyberpsychol Behav Social Networking. 2016;19(8):502–9.
41. Brent DA, McMakin DL, Kennard BD, Goldstein TR, Mayes TL, Douaihy AB. Protecting adolescents from self-harm: a critical review of intervention studies. J Am Acad Child Adolescent Psychiatry. 2013;52(12):1260–71.
42. Joshi SV, Hartley SN, Kessler M, Barstead M. School-based suicide prevention: content, process, and the role of trusted adults and peers. Child Adolescent Psychiatric Clin. 2015;24(2):353–70.
43. Dyson MP, Hartling L, Shulhan J, Chisholm A, Milne A, Sundar P, et al. A systematic review of social media use to discuss and view deliberate self-harm acts. PloS One. 2016;11(5):e0155813.
44. Lonergan A, Moriarty A, McNicholas F, Byrne T. Cyberbullying and internet safety: a survey of child and adolescent mental health practitioners. Irish J Psychol Med. 2021:1–8.

Virtual Mental Health and Telepsychiatry: Opportunities and Challenges with Pediatric Patients

11

Jeffrey Anderson

Introduction

Definition

Telemedicine is the practice of using technology to deliver healthcare when a provider and patient are in different places. Telemedicine can be delivered at a distance through technologies including telephone, email, mobile applications, and web-based systems. Telepsychiatry is a subtype of telemedicine and includes services delivered by a psychiatrist, such as evaluations, medication management, individual therapy, group therapy, and family therapy [1, 2]. It is typically synchronous, with two-way, real-time communication between a provider and patient, and it is conventionally performed by a live video appointment with a patient and psychiatrist [3]. Telepsychiatry can also be asynchronous, or delayed, which is telehealth technology that promotes sharing of healthcare by viewing recordings of clinical care and using patient portals, websites, and remote patient monitoring [4].

Setting

Telepsychiatry is used in a variety of settings, including outpatient clinics, emergency rooms, hospitals, correctional facilities, and schools. It is also used in a home-based setting, where the patient is at their home for the appointment [5]. Telepsychiatry for children and adolescents most commonly occurs in the outpatient setting [6].

J. Anderson (✉)
Department of Child and Adolescent Psychiatry, New York Presbyterian-Weill Cornell
Medical College, New York, NY, USA
e-mail: jba9005@nyp.org

© The Author(s), under exclusive license to Springer Nature Switzerland AG 2023
A. Spaniardi, J. M. Avari (eds.), *Teens, Screens, and Social Connection*,
https://doi.org/10.1007/978-3-031-24804-7_11

History of Virtual Mental Health and Telepsychiatry

Background

Telepsychiatry has its origins in the 1950s, with the University of Nebraska being the first program to use live interactive video conferencing for psychiatric treatment, consultation, and education. Other telepsychiatry programs existed throughout the late twentieth century, and in the early 2000s, the U.S. Department of Veterans Affairs began to offer telepsychiatry services [2]. In the past decade, there has been a large increase in the use of telehealth services in the United States [7].

Telepsychiatry and the COVID-19 Pandemic

Although telepsychiatry services have been available in certain locations for decades, the COVID-19 pandemic accelerated interest and use of telepsychiatry services [8]. Due to the need for physical distancing, regulatory changes were made during this public health emergency to maintain and expand access to psychiatric services. Flexibilities around medical licensure were enacted, and expansion and relaxation of telehealth regulations occurred in many states.

The American Psychiatric Association completed a survey in June 2020 and January 2021. Results showed a major shift to the use of telepsychiatry. The nearly 600 respondents to the initial survey worked in a variety of settings, from community clinics, group practice, solo practice, inpatient settings, and academic medical centers. Most respondents were not using telehealth prior to the COVID-19 pandemic, as 64% reported seeing zero patients via telepsychiatry; survey results from January 2021 showed 81% of respondents seeing the majority of their patients via telepsychiatry, with 94% of these patients being seen at their home during the appointment. Patient no-show rates dropped, and patients were satisfied with telepsychiatry for treatment and were more likely to continue with their course of treatment. As of January 2021, 64% of respondents treated patients across state lines, and three quarters of these respondents were not treating out-of-state patients before the pandemic [9].

Current State of Virtual Mental Health and Telepsychiatry

While telepsychiatry has been a useful way to provide psychiatric services while maintaining social distance and reducing COVID-19 transmission, it also has potential to continue when social distancing is no longer required. Multiple commercial vendors now provide telepsychiatry services, and many states are now considering implementing more permanent telepsychiatry policies [10].

Coverage for Telepsychiatry Services

In the United States, individual states can decide to cover Medicaid services provided via telepsychiatry. States determine which services to cover, where telepsychiatry services can be utilized, who can deliver telepsychiatry services, and reimbursement rates. For example, states have flexibility to reimburse telepsychiatry by telephone and/or video technology [8, 10]. States vary widely in regulation and definition of telepsychiatry, and no two states are the same [11]. Despite differences between states, all fifty states and the District of Columbia do provide live telepsychiatry video reimbursement through Medicaid. Twenty-two states reimburse for audio-only telephone appointments in some capacity. While audio-only telephone delivery has rarely been an acceptable modality for delivering telehealth services, that has been changing due to the COVID-19 pandemic; audio-only visits reach patients without access to broadband Internet for live videoconferencing [11, 12]. Many state Medicaid programs still limit qualifying originating sites for telepsychiatry appointments, often excluding a home site from reimbursement [12]. Private insurers frequently follow Medicaid in determining allowable services and situations [2].

Benefits of Virtual Mental Health and Telepsychiatry

Cost

Telepsychiatry can be a cost-effective alternative to traditional in-person appointments [3]. It is more convenient, readily accessible, and can reduce transportation costs when patients remain at home for appointments.

Benefit for Youth and Families

Telepsychiatry can be a good fit for youth. Patients are becoming more and more accustomed to technology in their daily lives and in healthcare, and youth especially have greater experience with and expectations of technology being present in their lives [2]. Multiple studies have shown that clinicians, parents, and young people rate high levels of satisfaction with telepsychiatry [6]. Telepsychiatry allows for a greater range of sites for treatment. Youth may feel less self-conscious and more able to talk about their feelings when appointments are conducted in their home, as this could potentially be a more comfortable setting. Appointments where the patient is at home also allow practitioners to observe patients in their living conditions [13]. School is another place where telepsychiatry services can allow a familiar setting and minimize disruption to classroom time and to parents' work [6]. Telepsychiatry is an alternative to families experiencing barriers to treatment, such as school activities and work, due to time being saved traveling to appointments. A psychiatrist is also able to see patients more frequently, for example, several times per week via telepsychiatry, whereas this may not be possible in a traditional format. Real-time urgent appointments for care are also possible. Additionally, telepsychiatry can improve the quality of care by disseminating expertise for specific psychiatric disorders [14]. For example, a psychiatrist with expertise in a specific disorder, such as obsessive-compulsive disorder, can reach a patient via telepsychiatry in an area where the patient may not have access to an expert in the disorder. There are no absolute contraindications for psychiatry other than the youth or parent refusing services in this format [15].

Improved Access and More Equitable Access

There is a severe shortage of psychiatrists in some areas of the United States, such as rural or remote areas. Telepsychiatry is a tool to address this need and improve access to care [16]. Access to child psychiatrists is especially a problem, with only half of children and adolescents with mental health needs receiving adequate treatment. Children and adolescents living outside of major cities are disproportionately affected by lack of access to a mental health specialist. Telepsychiatry can address the maldistribution of child and adolescent psychiatrists and allow patients in rural areas to be given treatment [15]. Additionally, telepsychiatry can help reach new populations in need of specialized care, such as treatment for tic disorders, substance use, and autism spectrum disorder [5]. Another benefit of telepsychiatry is that a patient in a rural area may feel uncomfortable receiving mental health treatment from a provider who lives in the rural area, because the patient may know the provider. Telepsychiatry addresses this by allowing the patient to see a provider that does not know them prior to the first encounter.

Evidence for Effectiveness

Telepsychiatry has proven to have effective outcomes in particular psychiatric conditions. Studies have focused on specific disorders within psychiatry and telepsychiatry, and a series of randomized clinical trials have shown equal outcome efficacy when compared to in-person treatments [6, 17]. One randomized trial found that treatment for obsessive-compulsive disorder in youth delivered via webcam was effective in reducing obsessive-compulsive symptoms [18]. Another randomized clinical trial studied telepsychiatry for the treatment of children with attention-deficit hyperactivity disorder (ADHD) that providing pharmacological treatment and caregiver behavior training; the telepsychiatry treatment was found to be an effective model to treat ADHD in communities with limited access to mental health services [4]. In regards to teletherapy, there are many studies involving youth that indicate that it is well tolerated [19, 20]. The American Psychiatric Association reports that telemedicine in psychiatry using video conferencing is an effective practice that increases access to care, and they support the use of it as a component of the mental health-care delivery system [1].

Challenges with Virtual Mental Health and Telepsychiatry

As telepsychiatry continues to grow, challenges become more apparent. Some challenges include establishing a therapeutic space for appointments, relative contraindications to telepsychiatry, community and cultural factors, and widening disparities in care. Figure 11.1 illustrates factors to consider when using telepsychiatry.

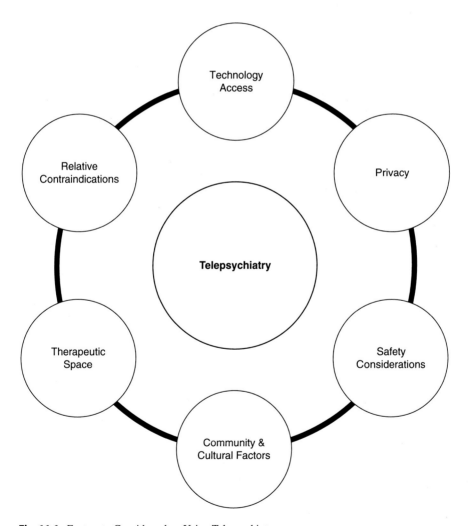

Fig. 11.1 Factors to Consider when Using Telepsychiatry

Establishing a Therapeutic Space

Psychiatrists should assess site appropriateness for telepsychiatry, including adequate space and visual and auditory privacy for patients. In addition to a secure Internet connection, an HIPAA-compliant platform for seeing the patient via video is needed. At the beginning of the appointment, it is important to confirm the identity and location of the patient, as well as confirm that the patient agrees to receive care via telepsychiatry. With children, there are additional considerations. The room may need to be large enough for a patient's parents or guardian to participate in the session. Another reason to consider space size is if the clinician needs to view a child patient's motor skills and activity. Parent involvement may be required to prepare for meetings and to minimize distractions in the room [6]. Determining a patient's willingness and ability to participate via video is necessary, and if the patient is not able or unwilling to do so, an appointment in-person should be considered.

Relative Contraindications

Although there are no absolute contraindications for telepsychiatry, there are some relative contraindications. A hostile home environment for children and adolescents, forensic evaluations, investigating allegations of abuse or neglect, family therapy with a history of interpersonal violence, and a volatile parent may not be suitable situations for telepsychiatry. In these situations, the child might not feel free to be honest in their environment. Some children with developmental disorders or disruptive behaviors might also not be able to tolerate telepsychiatry [15]. Children may also struggle with engaging in telepsychiatry and require adult supervision, which can affect the therapeutic relationship between a patient and psychiatrist. Additionally, a psychiatrist may need to obtain the weight and vital signs of a patient, which may not be possible with telepsychiatry. This issue can be mitigated by a parent or guardian obtaining weight and vital signs for the psychiatrist, or the patient periodically coming into an office for an appointment.

Community and Cultural Factors

Psychiatrists often differ in race, ethnicity, or culture from the patients and families they serve through telepsychiatry. Because the psychiatrist will likely reside at a distance from the patient site, it might be difficult to become familiar with the community's values, culture, and resources [15]. It is important for the psychiatrist to have an understanding of these factors.

Safety Considerations

Another consideration of using telepsychiatry from a distance is that not all communities have the same availability of crisis care, especially for children and

11 Virtual Mental Health and Telepsychiatry: Opportunities and Challenges...

adolescents and in underserved communities. Patients may have crises such as having episodes of self-harm, reporting suicidal or homicidal ideation, or being abused or neglected. Therefore, prior to establishing telepsychiatry services, psychiatrists should establish guidelines and procedures for a potential crisis using local community resources [6]. These resources may include a local EMS number and relevant local and national agencies' contact information.

As a psychiatrist is not physically in the room during an appointment using telepsychiatry, other safety preparations should be made, especially when seeing children or adolescents. These safety preparations may include confirming the time of the appointment with the parent or guardian and requesting that they be available or home during the session.

Telepsychiatry and the Digital Divide

Despite greater access in some areas using telehealth, some rural or underserved populations may experience a widening disparity in access because of the digital divide. The digital divide is the racial or socioeconomic access to digital resources, such as the Internet [21]. One of the key requirements for successful telehealth visits, particularly video visits, is access to high-speed (broadband) Internet. Approximately 100 million Americans do not subscribe to broadband Internet, with approximately 19 million Americans (6 percent of the population) not having access to fixed broadband service at speeds necessary for telepsychiatry appointments. Rural areas in particular lack access, and 14.5 million Americans without fixed broadband service live in these areas [22]. Telepsychiatry may not be suitable for these millions without broadband Internet, as it would not be possible to have synchronous video conferencing. In addition to access to broadband Internet, patients must have an Internet-capable device, such as a laptop or a smartphone. Patients and families must also have technology literacy to utilize telehealth services [13]. Table 11.1 lists questions to ask patients and their families prior to engaging in telepsychiatry (see Table 11.1) [21].

Table 11.1 Questions to ask patients and their families prior to engaging in telepsychiatry

Technology considerations	• Do you have access to high-speed broadband Internet? • Do you have access to an Internet-capable device, such as a smartphone, tablet, or laptop? • Does the device allow you to connect via video? • Do you know how to use the device? • Is audio-only telepsychiatry an option?
Therapeutic space considerations	• Is there a private space for sessions? • Is the room large enough to accommodate the patient, parent/guardian, or other family members, if needed? • Are there any distractions in the room that may need to be minimized?
Safety considerations	• Will the parent/guardian be present during the session? • If the parent/guardian is not present in the session, will they be present in the home during the session? • Does the parent/guardian have the local EMS number in case of emergency?

Considerations for the Psychiatrist

In addition to assessing site appropriateness for telepsychiatry, psychiatrists have other considerations, such as learning skills for engaging patients in telepsychiatry and assessing patient engagement in telepsychiatry. Engagement in telepsychiatry for the provider and patient includes showing up to appointments on time, staying on camera if the appointment is by video, and maintaining eye contact. Using props to engage patients, such as action figures, stuffed animals, and dolls, may be necessary for some patients. Integrating movement, such as dance, or including interactive activities may also help engage patients. Psychiatrists should make sure they have the proper licensure to deliver care via telepsychiatry, for example, if the patient is located in another state. Lastly, a psychiatrist should minimize distraction in their office as well, and should consider self-care issues that may arise with telepsychiatry, such as computer eye strain or the possible tendency to overwork.

Conclusion

During the COVID-19 pandemic, the utilization of telepsychiatry increased as a means to continue psychiatric services while limiting exposure to the virus. State regulations were loosened to allow telehealth, and some of these measures are being made permanent. Policies and regulations are continually evolving. Current limited research suggests that telepsychiatry is effective, but more research is needed to understand the best uses of telepsychiatry with children and adolescents. With more evidence and research, increasing guidelines, tools, and best practices will emerge. Additionally, as the use of telepsychiatry expands, we are increasingly understanding its limitations. Telepsychiatry offers the opportunity for psychiatrists to reach populations and communities that traditionally may not have access to psychiatric care. A key focus regarding telepsychiatry in the future should involve narrowing inequalities in access to care and addressing the digital divide.

Multiple Choice Questions
1. Telepsychiatry can be used in which of the following settings?
    A. Correctional facilities
    B. Emergency departments
    C. Elementary schools
    D. All of the above
       Correct Answer: D
2. Telepsychiatry is always a superior option for patients compared to in-person appointments.
    A. True
    B. False
       Correct Answer: B
3. You are a clinician working in a city and are preparing to deliver telepsychiatry services to an adolescent patient in a rural area in the same state. Which of the

following is NOT an appropriate question to ask the patient and family prior to engaging in telepsychiatry.

A. Do you have access to high-speed broadband Internet?
B. Is there a private space that the patient can use during appointments?
C. Will the patient's parent/guardian be secretly listening to the patient in another room during sessions?
D. Will the patient's parent/guardian be present during appointments?

Correct Answer: C

References

1. What is telepsychiatry? [Internet]. Washington: American Psychiatric Association; 2022 [cited 2022 Jul 11]. https://psychiatry.org/patients-families/telepsychiatry
2. Shore J. The evolution and history of telepsychiatry and its impact on psychiatric care: current implications for psychiatrists and psychiatric organizations. Int Rev Psychiatry. 2015;27(6):469–75. Epub 2015 Sep 23.
3. Telemedicine [Internet]. Baltimore (MD): Centers for Medicare & Medicaid Services; [cited 2022 Jul 11]. https://www.medicaid.gov/medicaid/benefits/telemedicine/index.html
4. Myers K, Vander Stoep A, Zhou C, et al. Effectiveness of a telehealth service delivery model for treating attention-deficit hyperactivity disorder: a community-based randomized controlled trial. J Am Acad Child Adolesc Psychiatry. 2015;54(4):263–74. Epub 2015 Jan 29.
5. Telepsychiatry [Internet]. Washington: American Academy of Child & Adolescent Psychiatry; 2022 [cited 2022 Jul 11]. https://www.aacap.org/aacap/Clinical_Practice_Center/Business_of_Practice/Telepsychiatry/Telepsych_Home.aspx
6. Gloff N, LeNoue S, Novins D, Myers K. Telemental health for children and adolescents. Int Rev Psychiatry. 2015;27(6):513–24. Epub 2015 Nov 5.
7. Fact sheet: telehealth [Internet]. [Chicago]: American Hospital Association; 2019 [cited 2022 Jul 11]. https://www.aha.org/system/files/2019-02/fact-sheet-telehealth-2-4-19.pdf
8. State Medicaid & CHIP telehealth toolkit: policy considerations for states expanding use of telehealth: COVID-19 Version [Internet]. [Baltimore]: Centers for Medicare & Medicaid Services; [cited 2022 Jul 11]. https://www.medicaid.gov/medicaid/benefits/downloads/medicaid-chip-telehealth-toolkit.pdf
9. Psychiatrists use of telepsychiatry during COVID-19 public health emergency: survey results [Internet]. [Washington]: American Psychiatric Association; 2021 Jul [cited 2022 Jul 11]. https://www.psychiatry.org/File%20Library/Psychiatrists/Practice/Telepsychiatry/APA-Telehealth-Survey-2020.pdf
10. State Medicaid & CHIP telehealth toolkit: policy considerations for states expanding use of telehealth: COVID-19 Version: Supplement # [Internet]. [Baltimore]: Centers for Medicare & Medicaid Services; 2021 Dec 6 [cited 2022 Jul 11]. https://www.medicaid.gov/medicaid/benefits/downloads/medicaid-chip-telehealth-toolkit-supplement1.pdf
11. State telehealth laws and Medicaid program policies: Fall 2021 [Internet]. [West Sacramento]: Public Health Institute/Center for Connected Health Policy; 2021 Oct [cited 2022 Jul 11]. https://www.cchpca.org/2021/10/Fall2021_ExecutiveSummary_FINAL.pdf
12. Policy trend maps [Internet]. West Sacramento (CA): Center for Connected Health Policy; 2022 [cited 2022 Jul 11]. https://www.cchpca.org/policy-trends/
13. Julien HM, Eberly LA, Adusumalli S. Telemedicine and the forgotten America. Circulation. 2020;142(4):312–4. Epub 2020 Jun 11.
14. Fortney JC, Pyne JM, Mouden SB, Mittal D, Hudson TJ, Schroeder GW, et al. Practice-based versus telemedicine-based collaborative care for depression in rural federally qualified health centers: A pragmatic randomized comparative effectiveness trial. Am J Psychiatry. 2013;170:414–25.

15. American Academy of Child and Adolescent Psychiatry Committee on Telepsychiatry and AACAP Committee on Quality Issues. Clinical update for telepsychiatry with children and adolescents. J Am Acad Child Adolesc Psychiatry. 2017;56(10):875–93. Epub 2017 Jul 25.
16. Severe shortage of child and adolescent psychiatrists illustrated in AACP workforce maps [Internet]. The American Academy of Child & Adolescent Psychiatry; 2022 [cited 2022 Jul 11]. https://www.aacap.org/AACAP/zLatest_News/Severe_Shortage_Child_Adolescent_ Psychiatrists_Illustrated_AACAP_Workforce_Maps.aspx
17. Hilty DM, Ferrer DC, Parish MB, Johnston B, Callahan EJ, Yellowlees PM. The effectiveness of telemental health: a 2013 review. Telemed J E Health. 2013;19(6):444–54.
18. Storch EA, Caporino NE, Morgan JR, et al. Preliminary investigation of web-camera delivered cognitive-behavioral therapy for youth with obsessive-compulsive disorder. Psychiatry Res. 2011;189:407–12. Epub 2011 Jun 17.
19. Nelson EL, Patton S. Using videoconferencing to deliver individual therapy and pediatric psychology interventions with children and adolescents. J Child Adolesc Psychopharmacol. 2016;26:212–20. Epub 2016 Jan 8
20. Nelson EL, Bui T. Rural telepsychology services for children and adolescents. J Clin Psychol. 2010;66:490–501.
21. Telepsychiatry and the digital divide [Internet]. Washington: American Psychiatric Association; 2022 [cited 2022 Jul 11]. https://www.psychiatry.org/psychiatrists/practice/telepsychiatry/ toolkit/digital-divide
22. Eighth broadband progress report [Internet]. Washington: Federal Communications Commission; [cited 2022 Jul 11]. https://www.fcc.gov/reports-research/reports/ broadband-progress-reports/eighth-broadband-progress-report

Lessons Learned from the COVID-19 Global Pandemic

12

Rakin Hoq and Aaron Reliford

Introduction

The COVID-19 pandemic has proven to be an unprecedented challenge for societies worldwide in multiple domains stretching far beyond the scope of mass infection. During the period of 2020–2021, the COVID pandemic resulted in over 5,000,000 deaths worldwide [1]. The highly transmissible nature of the illness has resulted not only in widespread infection and death, but subsequent mass closure of businesses, schools, and other public services. The cascading result of this pandemic has caused widespread grief for families and children, in addition to severely limiting socialization, limiting access to health-care services and other essential public services for many families, and furthermore magnified existing racial and economic disparities in societies throughout the world. The cumulative impact of many of COVID-19's downstream effects has complicated the mental health and mental healthcare for children and adolescents. This chapter will review the changes observed in the mental health and mental healthcare of children and adolescents over the course of the COVID-19 pandemic to date, and how the various aforementioned sequelae of the pandemic have affected children and families.

R. Hoq (✉)
Division of Child & Adolescent Psychiatry, Department of Psychiatry & Behavioral Sciences, Medical University of South Carolina, Charleston, SC, USA
e-mail: hoq@musc.edu

A. Reliford
Department of Child and Adolescent Psychiatry, NYU Child Study Center, NYU Grossman School of Medicine, New York, NY, USA

© The Author(s), under exclusive license to Springer Nature Switzerland AG 2023
A. Spaniardi, J. M. Avari (eds.), *Teens, Screens, and Social Connection*,
https://doi.org/10.1007/978-3-031-24804-7_12

Impacts on Mental Illness and Mental HealthCare During COVID-19 Pandemic

The COVID-19 pandemic has exacerbated an already existing mental health crisis among youth. Rates of depression and suicide in the pediatric population had already risen dramatically in the last 20 years, with rates of suicide in youth ages 10–14 tripling just between 2007 and 2017 alone [2, 3]. Since the COVID-19 pandemic started, children's mental health has suffered a massive setback overall. The worldwide prevalence of depression and anxiety in children has dramatically increased even further to now affecting 1 in 4 children and 1 in 5 children, respectively, which is a doubling of prepandemic estimates [4]. In comparison to 2019 (prepandemic), in 2020, when the pandemic struck worldwide, there was also a substantial increase in the overall proportion of pediatric emergency visits related to mental health crises in the United States, and in certain periods of the year, there was even a doubling of cases of suicide attempts presenting to pediatric emergency departments [5, 6]. In France, there was similarly an observed doubling of suicide attempts in children/adolescents between fall/winter of 2019 and winter of 2020 during their national lockdown, reflecting that the mental health crisis afflicting children was a worldwide one [7].

Depression, anxiety, and suicidal behaviors are not the only childhood mental health issues that have been significantly exacerbated by the pandemic though. In one study examining psychiatric admissions related to psychosis in children, there was a 66% increase observed in admissions due to psychosis compared to prepandemic rates [8]. While it is highly likely that pandemic-related circumstances including social isolation and decrease of access to services contributed to psychotic decompensations, there have also been multiple case reports published of psychosis suspected to be induced by COVID infections both in adults and adolescents. Theoretic mechanisms have been proposed for how COVID could induce psychosis: COVID may directly infect neurons in the brain, or cause systemic inflammation including in the central nervous system, or even potentially cause a post-infectious autoimmune syndrome that could explain subsequent psychotic reactions for some patients [9].

Similar to data assessing psychosis during the pandemic, in a systematic review of studies reviewing pediatric hospital admissions related to eating disorders, pooled data demonstrated an 83% increase in hospital admissions for pediatric eating disorders compared to prepandemic rates [10]. In this review, it was found in several studies that feelings of isolation and increased anxiety and depressive feelings contributed to exacerbations of adolescent eating disorder symptoms. To complicate this crisis further, there were mass closures of eating-disorder-focused treatment centers, so when children with severe eating disorders would be stabilized from medical hospitalizations, the step-down treatment options were limited or completely inaccessible.

Children with neurodevelopmental conditions like autism and ADHD also have been shown to suffer significantly under pandemic-related circumstances. Review of studies assessing behavioral disturbances in children with autism have showed

12 Lessons Learned from the COVID-19 Global Pandemic

significantly increased rates of reported aggressive behavior, and even worsening of communication [11]. Several factors were considered as contributing factors for these exacerbations including the closing down of many essential supportive services for special needs children in addition to the loss of structured schedules and supports offered by schools with nationwide school closures. Children with ADHD have been affected in many ways by pandemic-related circumstances. Review of the literature from the early onset of the pandemic and mass closures reflected worsening core ADHD symptoms like inattention and hyperactivity/impulsivity, in addition to worsening of mood symptoms and mood dysregulation [12]. These findings correlated with school closures and related social isolation and loss of supportive educational services. Importantly, it was also noted that externalizing behaviors, like aggressive outbursts, appeared to correlate with parental mood state-referring to parent stress.

Among other childhood psychiatric conditions that have been exacerbated during the pandemic, children with obsessive-compulsive disorder (OCD) have been observed to experience significant worsening of their OCD symptoms after onset of the pandemic as well [13] particularly with those having symptoms related to contamination with washing and cleaning rituals.

This increase in mental health crises has inevitably translated to psychiatric hospitalizations for children as well, with reports by some children's hospitals that upward of 53% of pediatric psychiatric admissions were related to COVID-19-related stressors over the course of 2020 [14]. The COVID-19 pandemic also rapidly shut down outpatient medical services, causing sudden and mass transition to telemedicine platforms for nearly all of outpatient health-care services. This was an effort to reduce exposure and infection risk from the COVID virus [15]. While this transition offered the benefit of a safer treatment format and for many added convenience, several barriers of telemedicine were exposed, including difficulty with maintaining confidentiality, especially for crowded households, and for many having limitations in access to the needed technology [16]. It is important to consider this change in mental health-care access as well as another contributing factor to exacerbation in crises and hospital admissions related to so many different illnesses as patients and families had lapses in their mental health-care services or delayed seeking treatment until their children's symptoms reached a high degree of severity, warranting hospital admission.

Direct Impact of COVID Infection and Death

COVID is attributed to over 5 million deaths worldwide, and in the United States alone has taken the lives of over 900,000 people. The effects of these individual deaths are not limited to simply lives lost, rather they are compounded exponentially on family and friends by bereavement. Bereavement of lives lost from COVID-19 is expected to affect millions of Americans. Children have been shown to be less susceptible to severe outcomes like hospitalization and death from the virus [17], but the adults in their lives have not shown the same resilience and made up the vast majority of COVID deaths. This left many children around the world suddenly without parental figures or other close adults and caregivers in their lives, forcing them into a state of grief unexpectedly [18]. By the beginning of the year 2021, there was a calculated 37,300 children that lost at least 1 parent to COVID just in the United States alone [19]. This sudden spike in parent death for children up to 17 years of age represented a nearly 20% increase in child bereavement. It is also important to note that among children affected, black and Hispanic children were disproportionately affected by parent death and bereavement (racial disparities will be discussed later in this chapter). Furthermore, during the peak of the pandemic, COVID-related deaths were frequent and often not handled gracefully with families as they occurred. One study in the U.K. found that in most cases of death and dying of a loved one from COVID-19, there was no discussion from a clinical professional with children of loved ones regarding the prognosis of their loved one. This was found to be a risk factor for maladjustment for children [20]. As COVID deaths occurred frequently, it is possible these described circumstances occurred often, leaving many children at a higher risk for complicated bereavement.

School Closure

The rapid spread of the COVID pandemic resulted in mass school closures across the globe as a public health effort to reduce community spread of infection. For most school systems, this was an unprecedented change, with educational systems largely left unprepared for a remote schooling approach. This resulted in prolonged periods of time with limited structure in school curriculums, and moreover a loss of socialization for children. It is known that prolonged social isolation is associated with higher rates of mental health issues for children and adolescents [21]. These research findings have been affirmed over the COVID pandemic as the children who have been subject to remote learning during this time have experienced a disproportionate rate of mental health problems [22]. In observational data of children's mental health in the United States alone, during lockdown periods of school closures, parents of children in primary education rated significant rises in behavioral, emotional, and attentional problems in their children during remote learning. There was a particular exacerbation of these issues in children in special education or with neurodevelopmental disorders like ADHD [23]. Similar findings have been replicated in other parts of the world as well, showing significant rises in rates of depressive symptoms among primary school students during school shutdowns [24].

School closures have also affected children by reducing overall physical activity and increasing screen time [25]. Children who have been subject to having higher rates of screen time have also been shown to be at higher risk of having more mental health issues. Conversely, children who have gotten more physical activity and had less screen time appeared to have better mental health outcomes [25]. Interestingly, mass school closures caused by the pandemic have also shed light on children's health in other ways besides harm. Remote schooling has generally resulted in later school start times and eliminated the time of travel. This consequently led to the observation of children sleeping longer, which may actually be considered a benefit of the remote schooling [26]. This may inform future adjustments to school start times to accommodate children's sleep needs, as it is known that early school start times frequently limit total sleep for children.

It is also important to emphasize that many children rely on school for essential health and support services, so in the midst of mass school closure, many children lost access to crucial mental health services as well. Over 50% of children receiving mental health services in the United States actually received some part of those services through school, with over 30% exclusively relying on school for those services [27]. The loss of the in-person school experience also resulted in loss of specialized and individualized education plans, severely impacting the learning experience of many children with mental disorders. For instance, children with autism requiring ABA therapy lost these critical support services before acclimation to virtual platforms, and children with ADHD requiring individualized education plans lost these accommodations, causing more anxiety and distress around learning [28]. On an even more fundamental level, schools are often a necessary resource of nutrition for many children through reduced or free lunch programs. During the quarantine, many students lost this necessary support in addition to falling into more unhealthy eating habits without the support of school cafeterias [28].

Impact of Economic Loss and Loss of Access to Essential Resources

Economic hardship, and loss of jobs among families worldwide, especially in the United States, has been a hallmark struggle of the pandemic. Parental job loss and economic hardship has invariably affected children. Firstly, these aforementioned circumstances have increased strain on parents. Consequently, increased parental stress has correlated to worsening of psychiatric symptoms for many children. Parents under excessive stress are at risk for not being able to attend to their children's needs as they would otherwise or engage in shared activities with their children as much. Moreover, the economic hardship for families caused by COVID-19 has directly resulted in housing instability, food insecurity, and limitation in children and family access to recreation, thereby destabilizing the lives of children and also limiting child wellbeing. With limited access to recreational activities both in school and in the community, many children had been left to turn mostly to their devices for recreational time. It has been shown that increased screen time during the pandemic lockdown was associated with depressive and anxiety symptoms, while less screen time and more family connectedness predicted better well-being for children [29].

The detrimental effects of parental job loss actually extend further than simply compromising child well-being or increasing mental health risk. It has been shown that job loss and housing instability are actually both risk factors for physical abuse to children [30]. Initially, with the onset of the pandemic, there was a substantial decrease in the number of child abuse cases reported. This was likely the consequence of children not being seen by usual mandated reporters such as their doctors or teachers during the extended period of pandemic-related lockdown. The reported cases being seen in this time have been reported to be of higher severity, and call centers have actually reported increased frequency of calls related to child abuse.

Earlier in this chapter, the mass school closures and initial shutdown of many essential clinical services were highlighted, but it is also important to emphasize the impact of the shutting down of support services for children with special needs. Children with neurodevelopmental disorders, such as autism, requiring additional support services, lost access to their essential supportive services such as applied behavioral analysis services, or even basic physical therapy, and occupational therapy resources [31]. These losses of support have left special needs children without critical supports to help their growth and development, and have also led to parents and caregivers suffering additional stress and anxiety as a result [32].

Racial Disparities Magnified by the Pandemic

The COVID pandemic has amplified challenges for youth from low-income families, and those from racial and ethnic minority groups. An increased burden of stressors through trauma, health disparities, and limited economic opportunities, faced by these youth prior to the pandemic, would certainly present greater risks for these youth during the pandemic [33]. Several studies and reports have highlighted the greater toll of COVID-related death and illness among racial and ethnic minority groups. One study early in the pandemic noted that over 4 thousand children experienced a parental or caregiver death due to COVID-19 (about 1 per 1000 children) and over 50% of these caregiver deaths were in three of New York City's boroughs with the most concentrated communities of black and Hispanic communities. Ultimately, Black and Hispanic children experienced parental/caregiver deaths from COVID-19 at twice the rate of Asian and white Children [34]. The study highlighted that wide racial/ethnic disparities in the rate of parental/caregiver deaths from COVID-19 was due to vast structural inequities that led to communities of color disproportionately being exposed to the virus.

Prior to the pandemic, it had become increasingly clear the toll of mental health of racial and ethnic minorities and those from impoverished backgrounds in the United States. For example, despite historically low levels of suicide, black children under 12 are now more likely to die by suicide than their white peers [35]. Additionally, by 2018, for black children, suicide was the 2nd leading cause of death for ages 10–14 and the third leading cause of death for ages 15–19 [36]. These factors, as well as the greater burden of stress on minority youth through increased prevalence of social determinants of health, would disproportionally put these youth at risk of mental health disparities as well.

Already, it has been shown that a large proportion of African-Americans who need mental healthcare don't receive mental healthcare [37], so prepandemic disparities in access to mental health services for these populations have likely been

12 Lessons Learned from the COVID-19 Global Pandemic

further exacerbated by the challenges of the covid pandemic [38]. In this context, despite the expectation of worsened mental health challenges for children and adolescents from minority backgrounds, data is lacking to show this challenge. Though one clear challenge that would potentially further serve the mental health burden in minority and low-income communities is the decreased access to mental health services typically available to these populations in schools due to mass school closure as discussed earlier in this chapter. Children from minority and impoverished communities have suffered greater challenges from being out of school due to having more limited access to a vital source of affordable and accessible medical and mental-health-care-school-based clinics [39]. This limited access has been further exacerbated by limited technological access to telemedicine-based care given inconsistent availability of resources such as computers and internet accessibility to minority communities, and continued stigmatization of engagement in mental health treatment [33, 39].

Telehealth and the New Health-Care Landscape Facilitated by COVID

Telehealth and telepsychiatry have been burgeoning in the health-care landscape for several years, but have progressed slowly due to several legislative roadblocks, which have varied widely from state to state. The onset of the COVID pandemic resulted in a sudden shutdown or reduction in health-care services in both the inpatient and outpatient settings in an attempt to limit spread of the virus. Many people were also limiting their engagement with health-care services out of fear of contracting the disease. This sudden shift in the health-care landscape forced the health-care system as a whole to turn to telehealth as a necessary solution to bridge the gaps and needs in care. What unfolded was expansion of reimbursement of telehealth services from Centers for Medicare and Medicaid Services (CMS) as well as for private payers, and loosening of reimbursement restrictions requiring face-to-face visits. These restrictions also loosened requirements for location of the patient as well as the provider. This allowed providers as well as patients to join virtual visits from their homes with the intention of minimizing travel and possible infectious exposure. The immense need for health-care services went as far as prompting a temporary allowance for telehealth services to be provided across state lines in certain states: for instance, providers of mental health services in New York were able to provide virtual mental healthcare to residents of neighboring states of New Jersey and Connecticut.

These changes have actually resulted in welcomed conveniences both for patients and providers. Multiple studies have now demonstrated that overall patient engagement in outpatient care has significantly increased since the widespread implementation of telemental health with visit cancellations and no show visits both reducing significantly [40]. Furthermore, there is evidence to support that children have widely received the transition to telehealth services favorably with a vast majority expressing feeling supported and finding care to be accessible [41]. It is notable though that for clinicians, the experience of the telehealth care experience has not been paralleled. The majority of clinicians in this same study found telehealth to either have no impact or even negative impact on the care experience, particularly, when it came to domains of providing care quality and meeting patient goals.

Since the initial emergency implementation of telehealth services, many mental health practices have gone entirely virtual both in the private practice landscape as well as institutional level for hospital and community mental health systems. As the COVID pandemic has gradually reached a point of relative stability with advents of effective vaccines and treatments, health-care policies have gradually tightened up again. This includes states are being more restrictive about telehealthcare being provided across state boundaries. These changes are gradually reeling in mental health-care access for many families who previously were relying on seeing providers in other states. As of now, telehealth appears to have been established as a new standard for providing mental healthcare at least in the outpatient setting with most practices at least allowing for a virtual option for care if not converting entirely to being telehealth practices.

Conclusion

The COVID-19 pandemic has not only taken the lives of millions of people worldwide, it has caused unexpected and unprecedented destabilization of several systems within society that normally provide fundamental scaffolding for the health and wellness of children. While children have had to face the inevitable challenges of sudden loss of caregivers and family members, this has been compounded by a breakdown of the educational system, sudden shifts in the mental health-care system and public health systems, and further disruption of their family systems through the effects of economic loss. These difficulties have all posed particular impact on children of black and Hispanic backgrounds. It is essential to factor in the complex interplay of these systems to appreciate the dynamic nature of children's mental health in the current era of the COVID pandemic.

Multiple Choice Questions
1. What have been the two mental illnesses that have increased the most in prevalence among children and adolescents since the beginning of the COVID-19 pandemic?
   A. Depression
   B. Anxiety
   C. Psychosis
   D. Eating Disorders
   E. A and B

   Correct Answer: E. Depression and anxiety are already the most common childhood mental illnesses by prevalence but have had a sharp increase in incidence over the pandemic lockdown. This has been related to several reasons including but not limited to extended isolation from peers, reduced access to recreational and also support resources, and increased parental/family strain due to the pandemic.

12 Lessons Learned from the COVID-19 Global Pandemic

2. What changes have been observed with child maltreatment during the pandemic?
   A. Childhood maltreatment cases have been reported more frequently.
   B. Childhood maltreatment cases have been reported less frequently.
   C. Childhood maltreatment cases reported have been of higher severity.
   D. B and C.

   Correct Answer: D. Childhood maltreatment during the pandemic lockdown was actually reported in less frequency, which is suspected to be related to reduced access to mandated reporters like teachers and doctors due to pandemic lockdown, but the reported cases seen during this time were seen to be of higher than normal severity.

3. Which of the following is true regarding disparities affecting black and Hispanic children over the course of the COVID-19 pandemic?
   A. Black and Hispanic children were affected by caregiver death at the same rate as non-Hispanic white children.
   B. Black and Hispanic children were affected by caregiver death at a disproportionately higher rate than non-Hispanic white children.
   C. Black and Hispanic children have had disproportionately less access to technological resources necessary for remote learning compared to non-Hispanic white children.
   D. Black and Hispanic children have had relatively equal access to technological resources necessary for remote learning compared to non-Hispanic white children.
   E. B and C

   Correct Answer: D. Mortality from the COVID-19 virus has disproportionately affected Black and Hispanic communities, which is related to a variety of pre-existing systemic disparities, leaving these ethnic groups seriously disadvantaged. This has subsequently left black and Hispanic children disproportionately affected by parent/caregiver death at a much higher rate compared to the non-Hispanic white population. Additionally, similar systemic disadvantages have been magnified with regards to access to resources over the course of pandemic lockdown with black and Hispanic children having significantly less access to needed technological recourses to participate in remote learning during mass school closure compared to non-Hispanic white children.

4. Over the course of pandemic-related lockdown with children suffering from eating disorders
   A. Fewer children have been hospitalized due to eating disorders compared to the year prior to onset of the COVID-19 pandemic.
   B. There was a significant rise in hospitalizations for children suffering from eating disorders during the pandemic compared to prepandemic rates.
   C. Outpatient eating disorder programs were largely unaffected by the pandemic.
   D. Many outpatient eating disorder programs were closed down, leaving treatment resources very limited for children suffering from eating disorders.
   E. B and d.

   Correct Answer: E. Children with eating disorders were uniquely affected by the pandemic, firstly by experiencing hardship with their mental health related to pandemic circumstances such as pervasive feelings of isolation and anxiety, which were reported to contribute to exacerbations in their eating disorders and lead to more frequent medically necessitated hospitalizations. In addition, eating disorder treatment services, which often rely on involved group and family based therapies, were shut down due to pandemic-lockdowns, leaving many children with inadequate access to needed treatment programs.

5. Which of the following accurately describes how children with autism have been affected by the COVID-19 pandemic?

A. Significant rises in behavioral disturbances such as aggressive behaviors were reported in children with autism over the course of the pandemic.

B. Essential support services like ABA therapies, occupational and physical therapy services were shut down due to the pandemic.

C. Many parents of children with autism developed increasing rates of anxiety over the course of the pandemic related to the limited resources and supports for their children.

D. All of the above.

Correct Answer: D. Children with autism have been at particular disadvantage due to pandemic circumstances. Children on the autism spectrum often rely significantly on tailored support services offered through school and the community to support their learning, functional, and behavioral needs, but due to mass closures of schools and also in-person therapies offered in communities, autistic children were suddenly left largely without any of these needed services and in turn there have been reports of significantly increased behavioral disturbances for autistic children at home, and increased rates of anxiety for parents of autistic children.

References

1. Coronavirus disease (COVID-19). Accessed February 18, 2022. https://www.who.int/emergencies/diseases/novel-coronavirus-2019?adgroupsurvey={adgroupsurvey}&gclid=CjwKCAiAx8KQBhAGEiwAD3EiP5TUIsC63REuXZ85Qs27DNwqxRh49PpEWb2G-IuR09RMedWhwlfpqhoCh_oQAvD_BwE

2. State suicide rates among adolescents and young adults aged 10–24 : United States, 2000–2018. Accessed February 18, 2022. https://stacks.cdc.gov/view/cdc/93667

3. Products - Data Briefs—Number 352—October 2019. Accessed February 18, 2022. https://www.cdc.gov/nchs/products/databriefs/db352.htm

4. Racine N, McArthur BA, Cooke JE, Eirich R, Zhu J, Madigan S. Global prevalence of depressive and anxiety symptoms in children and adolescents during COVID-19: a meta-analysis. JAMA Pediatr. 2021;175(11):1142–50. https://doi.org/10.1001/JAMAPEDIATRICS.2021.2482.

5. Leeb RT, Bitsko RH, Radhakrishnan L, Martinez P, Njai R, Holland KM. Mental health–related emergency department visits among children aged <18 years during the COVID-19 pandemic—United States, January 1–October 17, 2020. MMWR Morb Mortal Wkly Rep. 2020;69(45):1675–80. https://doi.org/10.15585/MMWR.MM6945A3.

6. Hill RM, Rufino K, Kurian S, Saxena J, Saxena K, Williams L. Suicide ideation and attempts in a pediatric emergency department before and during COVID-19. Pediatrics. 2021;147(3). https://doi.org/10.1542/PEDS.2020-029280.

7. Cousien A, Acquaviva E, Kernéis S, Yazdanpanah Y, Delorme R. Temporal trends in suicide attempts among children in the decade before and during the COVID-19

12 Lessons Learned from the COVID-19 Global Pandemic

pandemic in Paris, France. JAMA Netw Open. 2021;4(10). https://doi.org/10.1001/JAMANETWORKOPEN.2021.28611.

8. Deren B, Matheson K, Cloutier P. Rate of adolescent inpatient admission for psychosis during the COVID-19 pandemic: a retrospective chart review. Early Interv Psychiatry. 2022; https://doi.org/10.1111/EIP.13316. Published online.

9. Watson CJ, Thomas RH, Solomon T, Michael BD, Nicholson TR, Pollak TA. COVID-19 and psychosis risk: real or delusional concern? Neurosci Lett. 2021;741:135491. https://doi.org/10.1016/J.NEULET.2020.135491.

10. Devoe J, Han A, Anderson A, et al. The impact of the COVID-19 pandemic on eating disorders: a systematic review. Int J Eating Disorders. 2022; https://doi.org/10.1002/EAT.23704. Published online.

11. Psychiatric disorders and symptoms in children and adolescents during the COVID-19 pandemic: a review hilmi kodaz. Published online 2021. https://doi.org/10.14744/ejmo.2021.14105

12. McGowan G, Conrad R, Potts H. Challenges with managing children and adolescents with adhd during the covid-19 pandemic: a review of the literature. J Am Acad Child Adolesc Psychiatry. 2020;59(10):S251. https://doi.org/10.1016/J.JAAC.2020.08.412.

13. Tanir Y, Karayagmurlu A, Kaya İ, et al. Exacerbation of obsessive compulsive disorder symptoms in children and adolescents during COVID-19 pandemic. Psychiatry Res. 2020:293. https://doi.org/10.1016/J.PSYCHRES.2020.113363.

14. Reece L, Sams DP. The impact of COVID-19 on adolescent psychiatric inpatient admissions. Clin Child Psychol Psychiatry. 2021. Published online.; https://doi.org/10.1177/13591045211030666.

15. Barney A, Buckelew S, Mesheriakova V, Raymond-Flesch M. The COVID-19 pandemic and rapid implementation of adolescent and young adult telemedicine: challenges and opportunities for innovation. J Adolescent Health. 2020;67(2):164–71. https://doi.org/10.1016/J.JADOHEALTH.2020.05.006.

16. Palinkas LA, de Leon J, Salinas E, et al. Impact of the COVID-19 pandemic on child and adolescent mental health policy and practice implementation. Int J Environ Res Public Health. 2021;18(18). https://doi.org/10.3390/IJERPH18189622.

17. Fischer A. Resistance of children to Covid-19. How? Mucosal Immunol. Published online 2020. https://doi.org/10.1038/s41385-020-0303-9

18. Verdery AM, Smith-Greenaway E, Margolis R, Daw J. Tracking the reach of COVID-19 kin loss with a bereavement multiplier applied to the United States. Proc Natl Acad Sci U S A. 2020;117(30):17695–701. https://doi.org/10.1073/PNAS.2007476117.

19. Kidman R, Margolis R, Smith-Greenaway E, Verdery AM. Estimates and projections of COVID-19 and parental death in the US. JAMA Pediatr. 2021;175(7):745–6. https://doi.org/10.1001/JAMAPEDIATRICS.2021.0161.

20. Rapa E, Hanna JR, Mayland CR, Mason S, Moltrecht B, Dalton LJ. Experiences of preparing children for a death of an important adult during the COVID-19 pandemic: a mixed methods study. BMJ Open. 2021;11(8). https://doi.org/10.1136/BMJOPEN-2021-053099.

21. Loades ME, Chatburn E, Higson-Sweeney N, et al. Rapid systematic review: the impact of social isolation and loneliness on the mental health of children and adolescents in the context of COVID-19. J Am Acad Child Adolesc Psychiatry. 2020;59(11):1218–1239.e3. https://doi.org/10.1016/J.JAAC.2020.05.009.

22. Hawrilenko M, Kroshus E, Tandon P, Christakis D. The association between school closures and child mental health during COVID-19. JAMA Netw Open. 2021;4(9). https://doi.org/10.1001/JAMANETWORKOPEN.2021.24092.

23. Creswell C, Shum A, Pearcey S, Skripkauskaite S, Patalay P, Waite P. Young people's mental health during the COVID-19 pandemic. Lancet Child Adolesc Health. 2021;5(8):535–7. https://doi.org/10.1016/S2352-4642(21)00177-2.

24. Zhang L, Zhang D, Fang J, Wan Y, Tao F, Sun Y. Assessment of mental health of Chinese primary school students before and after school closing and opening during the COVID-19 pandemic. JAMA Netw Open. 2020;3(9). https://doi.org/10.1001/JAMANETWORKOPEN.2020.21482.

25. Tandon PS, Zhou C, Johnson AM, Gonzalez ES, Kroshus E. Association of children's physical activity and screen time with mental health during the covid-19 pandemic. JAMA Netw Open. 2021;4(10). https://doi.org/10.1001/JAMANETWORKOPEN.2021.27892.
26. Lim MTC, Ramamurthy MB, Aishworiya R, et al. School closure during the coronavirus disease 2019 (COVID-19) pandemic—impact on children's sleep. Sleep Med. 2021;78:108–14. https://doi.org/10.1016/J.SLEEP.2020.12.025.
27. Golberstein E, Wen H, Miller BF. Coronavirus disease 2019 (COVID-19) and mental health for children and adolescents. JAMA Pediatr. 2020;174(9):819–20. https://doi.org/10.1001/JAMAPEDIATRICS.2020.1456.
28. Hoofman J, Secord E. The effect of COVID-19 on education. Pediatr Clin North Am. 2021;68(5):1071–9. https://doi.org/10.1016/J.PCL.2021.05.009.
29. McArthur BA, Racine N, McDonald S, Tough S, Madigan S. Child and family factors associated with child mental health and well-being during COVID-19. Eur Child Adolesc Psychiatry. 2021;1:1–11. https://doi.org/10.1007/S00787-021-01849-9/TABLES/4.
30. Molnar BE, Scoglio AAJ, Beardslee WR. Community-level prevention of childhood maltreatment: next steps in a world with COVID-19. Int J Child Maltreat. 2021;3(4):467–81. https://doi.org/10.1007/S42448-020-00064-4.
31. Baweja R, Sierra, Brown L, Edwards EM, Murray MJ. COVID-19 pandemic and impact on patients with autism spectrum disorder. J Autism Dev Disord. 2022;52:473–82. https://doi.org/10.1007/s10803-021-04950-9.
32. Manning J, Billian J, Matson J, Allen C, Soares N. Perceptions of families of individuals with autism spectrum disorder during the COVID-19 crisis. J Autism Dev Disord. 1234;51:2920–8. https://doi.org/10.1007/s10803-020-04760-5.
33. Cortés-García L, Hernández Ortiz J, Asim N, et al. COVID-19 conversations: a qualitative study of majority Hispanic/Latinx youth experiences during early stages of the pandemic. Child Youth Care Forum. 2021. Published online.; https://doi.org/10.1007/S10566-021-09653-X.
34. Brundage S, Ramos-Callan K. COVID-19 ripple effect the impact of COVID-19 on children in New York state part 1: death of parent or caregiver. Published online 2020.
35. Bridge JA, Horowitz LM, Fontanella CA, et al. Age-related racial disparity in suicide rates among US youths from 2001 through 2015. JAMA Pediatr. 2018;172(7):697–9. https://doi.org/10.1001/JAMAPEDIATRICS.2018.0399.
36. Mental and behavioral health—African Americans—the office of minority health. Accessed February 28, 2022. https://minorityhealth.hhs.gov/omh/browse.aspx?lvl=4&lvlid=24
37. McGuire TG, Miranda J. New evidence regarding racial and ethnic disparities in mental health: policy implications. Health Aff (Millwood). 2017;27(2):393–403. https://doi.org/10.1377/HLTHAFF.27.2.393.
38. Saltzman LY, Lesen AE, Henry V, Hansel TC, Bordnick PS. COVID-19 mental health disparities. https://home.liebertpub.com/hs. 2021;19(S1):S5–S13. https://doi.org/10.1089/HS.2021.0017
39. Torres-Pagán L, Terepka A. School-based health centers during academic disruption: challenges and opportunity in urban mental health. Psychol Trauma. 2020;12:S276–8. https://doi.org/10.1037/TRA0000611.
40. Eyllon M, Ben BJ, Daukas K, Fair M, Nordberg SS. The impact of the Covid-19-related transition to telehealth on visit adherence in mental health care: an interrupted time series study. Administration Policy Mental Health Mental Health Services Res. 2022;49(3):453–62. https://doi.org/10.1007/S10488-021-01175-X/TABLES/3.
41. Nicholas J, Bell IH, Thompson A, et al. Implementation lessons from the transition to telehealth during COVID-19: a survey of clinicians and young people from youth mental health services. Psychiatry Res. 2021;299. https://doi.org/10.1016/J.PSYCHRES.2021.113848.

Index

A
American Academy of Child and Adolescent Psychiatry (AACAP), 147, 148
American Academy of Pediatrics (AAP), 2, 147
Anonymity, 36, 53
Anxiety disorders, 137, 138
Attention-deficit/hyperactivity disorder (ADHD), 126, 127, 169
Attribution theory, 41

C
Caregivers, 138, 142
Catfishing, 52
Child Behavior Checklist, 3
Child development, 7
Children's Online Privacy Protection Act (COPPA), 145, 146
Common Sense Media, 52
Compulsive sexual behavior disorder (CSBD), 124
Confidentiality, 23–24
COVID-19 pandemic, 136, 137, 158, 175, 176
  child maltreatment, 175
  eating disorders, 175
  economic loss, 171, 172
  hospitalization and death, 169, 170
  loss of access to resources, 171, 172
  mental health care, 168, 169
  mental illness, 168, 169, 174
  racial disparities, 172, 173
  school closure, 170, 171
  telehealth, 173, 174
  telepsychiatry, 173, 174
Cyberbullying, 18, 21, 22, 24, 35, 68, 87, 149, 150
  cyber-aggression, 80, 82
  definition, 79
  demographic risk factors
    age, 89, 90
    gender, 90, 91
    minority youth, 91, 92
  fraping, 98
  mental health, 92, 93
  parenting challenges
    internet usage, 95, 96
    parental supervision and safety, 94
    recommendations, 96–98
    resources, 95
    screen time and online content, 94
    warning signs, 95
  perpetration risk, 88, 89
  prevalence, 84–86
  protective factors, 93, 94
  social media, 83, 84
  vs. traditional bullying, 82, 83
  victimization risk, 87, 88
Cyberstalking, 18

D
Depression
  adolescent, 63–65
  exercise, 70, 71
  internet use, 65
  multitasking, 70
  personal characteristics
    age differences, 68, 69
    gender differences, 68
    personality differences, 69
  sleep, 70
  social media
    Facebook depression, 71
    feedback, 66, 67
    FOMO, 72
    friends *vs.* strangers, 67
    MOST model, 73
    passive *vs.* active, 66
    SOVA, 73

© The Editor(s) (if applicable) and The Author(s), under exclusive license to Springer Nature Switzerland AG 2023
A. Spaniardi, J. M. Avari (eds.), *Teens, Screens, and Social Connection*,
https://doi.org/10.1007/978-3-031-24804-7

Developmental disabilities, 138
Digital advertising, 145
Digital Divide, 163
Digital footprint, 39
Digital literacy, 146, 153
Digital media exposure, 2
Digital technology, 2, 4, 5, 8
Digital world and identity, 52

E
Education, 42, 43
Encountering triggering content, 36, 37
Encouraging high risk behaviors, 37
Erikson's stages of Psychosocial
Development, 50, 51
Exercise, 70, 71

F
Facebook, 12, 14, 15, 31, 52, 71, 74
Fake Instagram (*finsta*), 52
Fear Of Missing Out (FOMO), 44, 71, 72
Federal Child Abuse Prevention and Treatment
Act (CAPTA), 23

G
Geosocial networking applications
(GNAs), 107
Group violence, 18

H
Harassment, 36

I
Identity, definition, 50
Identity expression, 57
Identity formation, 57
Impersonating and account forgery, 18
Impression management, 54
Instagram, 12, 14–16, 18–22, 24, 25, 31,
34, 52, 54
Internet Gaming Disorder (IGD), 128
biopsychosocial variables, 116
diagnostic criteria, 114–116
Diagnostic Questionnaire (DQ), 114
patient history, 126, 127
pornography, 123–125
recommendations
for clinicians, 128
for parents, 121, 122

risk and protective factors, 118, 119
screening, 117–119
social media, 122, 123
treatment and prevention, 120, 121
tree-based model, 116
video streaming, 125
withdrawal phenomenon, 117
Internet safety, 153
clinicians role, 148–151
federal law, 153
parents role, 146–148
patient history, 151, 152
Interpersonal connection, 31, 39

L
Lesbian Gay Bisexual Transgender Queer Plus
(LGBTQ+) youth, 55–57, 139

M
Major depressive disorder, 64
Marcia's identity statuses, 51
Media use, 2, 4, 5, 7
Mental health professionals, 57
Moderated online social therapy (MOST)
model, 73
Mood disorders, 137, 138
Movement disorders, 138
Multitasking, 70

N
Neuroscience-backed technology, 6
Non-suicidal self-injurious behavior
(NSSIB), 19, 20

O
Obsessive-compulsive disorder (OCD), 169
Online communities for adolescents
patient history, 140, 141
social media
COVID-19 pandemic, 136, 137
developmental disabilities, 138
LGBTQ+ population, 139
mental health, 136
mood and anxiety disorders, 137, 138
movement disorders, 138
online gaming communities, 139, 140
online political activism, 140
recommendations to parents, 140
Online disinhibition, 36
Online forums (Reddit), 52

Index

Online gaming community, 139, 140, 142
Online political activism, 140
Online supervision, 57
Online world identity, minority youth, 53, 54

P

Parental report, 22
Parental screen time, 5
Parent mobile technology, 5
Photo filters, 52
Pornography, 123–125
Profile, 52
Psychodynamic therapy, 57

R

Random Intercept Cross-lagged Panel
    Modeling, 118
Real world identity, minority youth, 53, 54

S

Screen time effect
    AAP guidelines, 2
    benefit, 6
    clinical considerations, 5
    cognitive development, 3
    impact of parental screen time, 5
    language development, 3, 4
    limitations, 4
    parental screen time, 5
    sleep, 4
    technology, 6
Self-esteem, 17, 54–55, 58
Self-harming behavior, 22
Selfies, 52
Self-presentation, 54
Sexting, 38, 150
    clinicians, 109
    experiences, 105
    gender differences, 106
    geosocial networking applications, 107
    legal implications, 109
    mental health concerns, 107, 108
    positive and negative outcomes, 105
    prevalence, 103, 104
    risky behavior, 108
    in younger adolescence, 104–107
Sexual harassment, 18
Sexually explicit information, 22
Sexual minority adolescents (SMA), 107
Sleep, 70
Snapchat, 12, 14, 15, 18–22, 24, 25, 31, 52

Social comparison theory, 39
Social connection, 32, 33
Social emotional well-being (SEWB)
    score, 17
Social media, 54, 142
    adolescents, 31–45
    advantages
        communication and social
            connection, 32, 33
        educational applications, 34
        exploring identity, creativity, and
            interests, 33, 34
        health information and resources, 34
        seeking, receiving, and providing social
            support, 33
    applications, 14, 15
    attribution theory, 41
    COVID-19 pandemic, 136, 137
    cyberbullying, 83, 84
    definition, 31, 82
    depression
        feedback, 66, 67
        friends *vs.* strangers, 67
        passive *vs.* active, 66
    detrimental effects, 17
    developmental disabilities, 138
    disadvantages
        communication, negative effects of, 37
        cyberbullying, 35
        digital footprint, 39
        encountering triggering content, 36, 37
        encouraging high risk behaviors, 37
        harassment, 36
        sexting, 38
    gender differences, 16
    IGD, 122, 123
    LGBTQ+ population, 139
    mental health, 136
    mood and anxiety disorders, 137, 138
    movement disorders, 138
    online gaming communities, 139, 140
    online political activism, 140
    origin, 31
    recommendations to parents, 140
    risk, 18
    screening, 20–23
    social comparison, 39
    teenage use of, 15, 16
    in therapy
        education, 42, 43
        identifying risks and encouraging
            positive use, 43, 44
Supporting Our Valued Adolescents
    (SOVA), 73

Index

T
Telehealth, 158, 173, 174
Telemedicine, definition, 157
Telepsychiatry, 164, 173, 174
    benefits, 159–161
    community and cultural factors, 162
    coverage, 159
    definition, 157
    Digital Divide, 163
    factors, 161
    HIPAA-compliant platform, 162
    history, 158
    in-person appointments, 164
    psychiatrist considerations, 164
    relative contraindications, 162
    safety, 162, 163
    settings, 157, 164
Teletherapy, 160
Tiktok, 11, 12, 14–16, 18, 20–22, 24, 25,
        32, 34, 68
Traditional bullying, 82, 83
Triggering content, 36

U
Unipolar depression, 63

V
Verbal violence, 18
Videoconferencing, 159
Video-on-demand (VOD), 125
Video streaming, 125
Virtual mental health, *see* Telepsychiatry
Visual violence, 18

W
WhatsApp, 14

Y
Youtube, 14, 16, 31, 34